Years of Change and Suffering

MODERN PERSPECTIVES ON CIVIL WAR MEDICINE

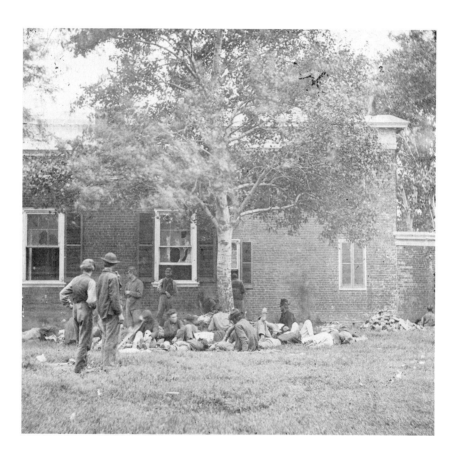

Wounded from the Battle of the Wilderness, May 1864
Source: Library of Congress

Years of Change and Suffering

MODERN PERSPECTIVES ON CIVIL WAR MEDICINE

James M. Schmidt and Guy R. Hasegawa
Editors

EDINBOROUGH PRESS

2009

Edinborough Press
P. O. Box 13790
Roseville, Minnesota 55113-2293
1-888-251-6336
www.edinborough.com

The book is set in Adobe Caslon Pro.

Cover image credits

Front cover: Wounded from the Battle of the Wilderness, Library of Congress.

Back cover: Patients in Ward K of Armory Square Hospital, Washington, D.C.,
Library of Congress.

LIBRARY OF CONGRESS CATALOGING-IN-PUBLICATION DATA
    Years of change and suffering : modern perspectives on Civil War medicine
/ James M. Schmidt and Guy R. Hasegawa, editors.
        p. cm.
    Includes bibliographical references and index.
    ISBN 978-1-889020-35-8 (casebound : alk. paper) — ISBN 978-1-889020-
36-5 (softbound : alk. paper)
    1. United States—History—Civil War, 1861-1865—Medical care. 2. Medi-
cine, Military—United States—History—19th century. I. Schmidt, James
M., 1964- II. Hasegawa, Guy R., 1952-.
    E621.Y436 2009
    616.9'8023—dc22
                        2009032801

Contents

Faithful, indeed, is the spirit that remembers
After such years of change and suffering!

Remembrance
Emily Brontë

Foreword

I thought I knew something about history. I took many history courses as an undergraduate. I even tutored fellow students in Western Civilization. The history of medicine was part of my specialty certification examination. I've published four books and a dozen articles on various aspects of nineteeth century medicine. To my surprise and delight, this book—*Years of Change and Suffering*—is full of things I hadn't known before.

For example, the great medical student migration on the eve of the Civil War was new to me. In 1859, hundreds of Southern boys—studying medicine in New York and Philadelphia—fled south to the Medical College of Virginia (MCV) in Richmond. The exodus was not a trickle, but a sudden and orchestrated surge. Before 1861, MCV was a relatively minor star in the galaxy of American medicine. The Civil War propelled the school to prominence as the Confederacy's leading center of medical education. The stresses of keeping students when the army was crying for men, funding a teaching hospital, overcoming inflation, and treating both soldiers and civilians, is a stirring story.

There were ironies. With death everywhere, the school still lacked corpses for the anatomy dissection laboratories as the school's long-term "resurrection man" (grave robber) quit and no new one could be found. The Yankee noose around Richmond and Petersburg continued to tighten and each day some new shortage or problem arose. As the end neared, the school was forced to sell its one horse, the one that pulled the ambulance. (If horses talked, what tales that faithful beast could tell!)

Another chapter approaches the Civil War through different eyes: those of the editors of *Scientific American* magazine. During the war, the magazine evolved into an idea exchange for new weapons, improved sanitation, and helpful hints for boys away from mother. *Scientific American* carried many articles detailing new surgical instruments, improved ambulances, better splints and prosthetics, and—in an apotheosis of inventiveness—a device to filter lizards out of drinking water. Sadly, knowledge of the danger of organisms far smaller than lizards lay in the future.

Other excellent chapters describe the life and contributions of the brilliant surgeon and administrator, J. J. Chisolm; the Confederate search for local botanicals to substitute for medicines no longer available because of the blockade; a detailed examination of urological wounds; the advances made in neurology by the extraordinary team of S. W. Mitchell, W. W. Keen, and G. R. Morehouse; and, a discussion of evolving views on amputation during the war. The final chapter on the mental health of veterans makes the point that our study of Civil War medicine should not end with the surrender at Appomattox.

There are, of course, many books about medical aspects of the Civil War: George W. Adams's *Doctors in Blue*, H. H. Cunningham's *Doctors in Gray*, and Alfred J. Bollett's *Civil War Medicine: Challenges and Triumphs*, stand out as the best surveys. Special studies include my and Jack D. Welsh's *Tarnished Scalpels*, which considered surgeons who faced discipline for medical incompetence and malfeasance; Robert E. Denney's *Civil War Medicine: Care and Comfort of the Wounded*, which took a chronological approach; and Margaret Humphreys's *Intensely Human*, which specifically explored the medical care of African-American soldiers.

Years of Change and Suffering adds a whole new dimension to the literature on Civil War medicine: it does not duplicate earlier work, but gives us in-depth treatment of subjects explored only minimally in other works and illuminates the quantum leap in medical knowledge and organization spawned by the vast necessities and cataclysmic suffering of a continent at war. This approach erases the gap between "then" and "now": medicine in our era reflects the fountainhead of Civil War innovation, a never-ceasing evolution that continues to this day.

My brief observations barely scratch the surface. This is a remarkable book. The contributors are the top people in their respective fields. The narrative prose is lively and clear. The editing is professional. I found it both informative and enjoyable.

Thomas P. Lowry, M.D.
Woodbridge, Virginia

Years of Change and Suffering

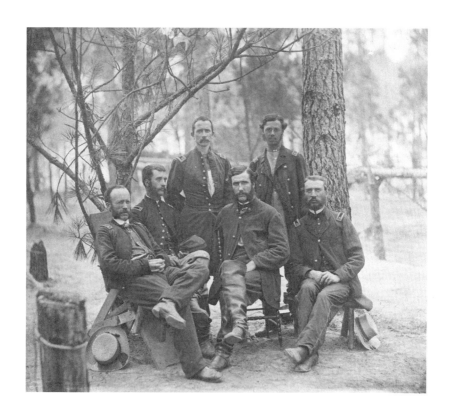

Union surgeons, Broadway Landing, Virginia
Source: Library of Congress

Introduction

Where does the story of Civil War medicine begin? For more than two hundred Southern students studying among Philadelphia's several medical colleges, it began with the hanging of abolitionist firebrand John Brown on December 2, 1859. Not only was Brown's execution a pivotal event in the road to disunion of the United States of America, the episode—and subsequent fisticuffs between abolitionists and Southerners in the "City of Brotherly Love"—proved to be the impetus for the students to "secede" and finish their studies at home, most at Richmond's Medical College of Virginia.

The press reacted to the episode with surprisingly mixed reporting on both sides of the Mason-Dixon Line. One Iowa paper declared that the "Southern 'deputy saw bones'" did "a very foolish thing, for the Philadelphia medical schools are the best in the United States." Another Northern paper—rejoicing at the departures—suggested that "300 ignorant doctors let loose in the South might be as destructive of life as a 'Brown Invasion.'" The *Lancaster Intelligencer*, however, found the Southern students "intelligent young men . . . universally esteemed by the great mass of our citizens," and thought them justly "indignant at the . . . mad fanatics of the North, especially those residing in Philadelphia."[1]

In Richmond, the *Enquirer* declared the exodus "Good News for Richmond and the South" and an "important step for building up our Medical College and aiding in the independence of the South." The *Richmond Whig*, though, railed against the city council for subsidizing the exodus with $5,000 to meet the extra expenses of the students, scoffed at the notion that the students were "constrained" to leave the North, and considered the whole affair "absurd and foolish." On December 22, 1859, the students arrived by train in Richmond, where they were greeted by "an immense throng of citizens . . . the shouts of the men were deafening, which the ladies manifested by the waving of their handkerchiefs."[2]

It is with the arrival of the students in Richmond that Jodi Koste begins "Medical School for a Nation," in which she describes the transformation of the Medical College of Virginia (MCV) from "a sleepy state institution into the premier medical school for the nascent Confederate nation." Drawing on substantial material from MCV's archives—of which she is the steward—she proposes that the school's location in the Confederate capital, a stable faculty, and a newly constructed hospital all helped to propel the college to a place of prominence, while other Southern medical schools were forced to close. More important, she argues that the school's war experience "gave the faculty chances to provide clinical instruction and undertake new professional activities," which—when combined with the traditional curriculum—enhanced the experience for the repatriated students and helped to "catapult MCV to 'first in the Confederacy.'"

Once the Civil War began in earnest, inventors on both sides of the Mason-Dixon Line set their minds and tools to work and—as one Northern newspaper declared—directed "their attention forthwith to the improvement of all sorts of instrumentalities." So confident was the paper in the preeminence of "Yankee ingenuity" that it predicted that Union masterminds would "produce some patent Secession-Excavator, some Traitor-Annhilator, some Rebel-Thrasher, some Confederate State Milling Machine, which will grind through, shell out, or slice up this war, as if it were a bushel of wheat or an ear of corn or a big apple."[3]

During the Civil War, *Scientific American*—America's oldest continuously published magazine—played an important role by fostering and reporting on inventions that had an impact on the battlefields and waters. Not surprisingly, wartime issues of *Scientific American* have been used as resources in modern studies of mid-nineteenth century military technology. In his contribution, "A Multitude of Ingenious Articles," Jim Schmidt—a chemist by training and profession—alerts readers to a lesser-known fact: *Scientific American* played an equally important role in fostering the "healing arts" by advising leaders how to maintain the health of the army and urging inventors to give attention to unmet medical needs. The magazine also reported on advances in medical technologies, including ambulances, medicines, and artificial arms and legs.

Schmidt acknowledges that it is "impossible to separate weaponry from medicine in the Civil War, as arms were responsible for hundreds of thousands of deaths and many more thousands of wounds on the battlefields," and readers will be surprised to see how weapons of the future, especially chemical and biological, began to emerge during the war. He also contends that study of *Scientific American*'s wartime pages supports recent historical scholarship in the economics and social impact of invention in the nineteenth century, including the increase in patenting activity by women, the danger of relying solely on patent counts as a measure of inventive activity, and the effect that professional ethics had in restricting patenting activity in the medical community.

One invention that had a tremendous impact on Civil War tactics *and* medicine was not a new one at all: the Minié bullet, introduced about fifteen years earlier by the French army officer Claude-Etienne Minié in the late 1840s. The "minnie ball"—as it was often referred to by soldiers—was not a ball at all, but rather a connoidal projectile that proved to be a powerful missile, indeed, when fired through a rifled barrel, Civil War surgeons quickly recognized from battlefield experience that the Minié was "much the more destructive" compared with the round ball fired from a smoothbore musket, a fact reinforced by very recent research using ordnance gelatin to examine the wound ballistics of the Minié. The force of the bullet caused tremendous injury to soft tissue and even worse damage when it struck bone, with amputation in such cases often offering the only chance of saving the life of a patient.[4]

It is ironic, then, that if asked to conjure up a picture of Civil War medical practice, many people today imagine callous surgeons indiscriminately hacking limbs off of soldiers whose only medication was a swig of whiskey. Even during the Civil War, the increasingly common sight of amputees led many citizens to conclude that limbs were being removed too often. Medical treatment, including amputation, has been called one of the Civil War's "most dismal failures," when in fact it was the most frequent major operative procedure that could be done successfully, and—contrary to popular belief—patients undergoing amputation were almost always anesthetized with chloroform or ether.[5]

Amputation is the topic of the chapter by Alfred Jay Bollet, author of the modern classic survey *Civil War Medicine: Challenges and Triumphs*. Dr. Bollet draws on his far-ranging expertise in medical history—and a distinguished career in clinical practice and medical education—to provide the proper context in which to consider amputations. Although there were concerns that many amputations were unneeded or incompetently performed, some expert observers of the time contended that more soldiers would have survived had the procedure been carried out more often. Dr. Bollet points out that care provided during the Civil War was sometimes superior to that rendered in the Crimean War and Franco-Prussian War, which occurred in the same era.

F. Terry Hambrecht's contribution about Confederate surgeon J. J. Chisolm continues the theme of innovation introduced in Jim Schmidt's chapter. While Chisolm is justly recognized for his editions of *A Manual of Military Surgery for Use of Surgeons in the Confederate Army*, Dr. Hambrecht adds to our current knowledge by drawing on previously unpublished material to characterize Chisolm as an innovator and man of action. Chisolm could hardly ask for a more fitting biographer than Dr. Hambrecht, who had a distinguished career as a director at the National Institutes of Health and pioneered research in prostheses for the neurologically disabled, including the blind, deaf, and paralyzed.

Dr. Hambrecht, a long-time researcher in Civil War medicine and an expert in Confederate medical personnel, shares his transcription of two letterbooks from 1861-1862 that show Chisolm constantly seeking to improve conditions for patients through his considerable skills as a physician, organizer, administrator, designer, inventor, and author. Chisolm treated sick and wounded soldiers, organized hospitals, served as a medical purveyor and director of a medical laboratory, invented or improved the design of medical apparatus, and wrote a major textbook used throughout the war by Confederate surgeons. He was not shy about making his frank opinions known to decision-makers, especially Confederate Surgeon General Samuel Preston Moore.

Dr. Hambrecht, in fact, considers Moore to be the only medical officer who might have matched Chisolm in improving Confederate medicine—high praise indeed for Chisolm, given the almost universal respect that historians have accorded Moore. Chisolm's contributions to medicine continued after the war, notably as a pioneer in the specialty of ophthalmology. In 1887, Chisolm examined the young Helen Keller, advising her father (also a Confederate veteran) to take her to Alexander Graham Bell, who in turn introduced the family to "Miracle Worker" Annie Sullivan. Chisolm's continued importance to the history of Civil War medicine is evident in the fact that he is mentioned or cited in three other chapters in this collection.

Wounds to the arms and legs, as described by Jay Bollet, were clearly not the only devastating injuries sustained by Civil War soldiers. Due to the nature of the fighting, soldiers sometimes fought kneeling, sitting, or lying prone, and they were exposed to being shot in the buttocks or genitals. In his contribution, "The Privates Were Shot," surgeon Harry Herr describes urological wounds and treatment. Dr. Herr combines statistics and case reports, largely from the *Medical and Surgical History of the War of the Rebellion*, with his knowledge of wartime surgical beliefs and practices to illustrate the enormous clinical challenges faced by caregivers and the dismal outcomes that patients were likely to experience.

Dr. Herr's case studies give graphic and grim witness to the debilitating nature of urethral wounds suffered by soldiers during the Civil War. Although generally not as fatal when compared with wounds of the chest or abdomen, urethral injuries were very troublesome for surgeons to treat, and survivors dealt with serious and painful consequences—physical and emotional—for the rest of their lives. Those consequences included chronic infection, constant leakage of urine, difficulty walking, and sexual dysfunction, as only a few examples.

The Civil War, states Dr. Herr, was a training ground for American clinicians, whose formal education was supposedly inferior to that of their European counterparts. Ironically, the survival rate was higher for Civil War than Crimean War casualties, a fact partially explained by how effectively Civil War surgeons learned from their clinical experience. Dr. Herr believes that European surgeons, reporting on their experiences in the Crimean War, had exaggerated the gravity of wounds to the pelvis. Mortality and morbidity of these types of injuries was actually better in the Civil War than the Crimean War, and Dr. Herr concludes that surgeons—North and South—must have been doing something right. He also points out that the eagerness of surgeons to share their recently acquired insight was evident in the postwar formation of medical societies, which helped to improve the quality of American medicine.

Maintaining the quality of care during the Civil War tested the resourcefulness of the South as it strove, in the face of an increasingly effective blockade, to supply its troops with medicines. Guy R. Hasegawa, a specialist in Civil War pharmacy and medical purveying, uses an array of primary source materials to describe how the Confederate Medical Department turned to internal resources—animal, vegetable, and mineral—to produce drugs. Hopes were high that medicines derived from Southern plants, in particular, would adequately fill in for standard drugs that were too scarce or expensive to purchase and issue in large quantities. Newspaper notices placed by medical officers called on citizens to collect native medicinal plants and deliver them to army-operated facilities for processing.

In examining the selection of plants to be gathered, Dr. Hasegawa questions the real influence of *Resources of the Southern Field and Forests*, a book credited by some historians with "maintaining the Southern war effort for many months longer than if it had not been written." A factor complicating the use of Southern flora was the reluctance of some medical personnel to use plant-based remedies that they associated with unconventional or fringe practitioners. Mined materials, such as sulfur and iron pyrites, were used in chemical processes necessary to manufacture ether and chloroform. Citizens even gathered potato flies, which were dried and ground for use as a blistering agent.[6]

The production of Southern drugs was spearheaded by Surgeon General Moore, whose belief in the vital role of native plants resembled, according to one observer, an obsession. Moore and his medical purveyors sought the cooperation of other organizations active in the war effort—-the Nitre and Mining Bureau and the Navy, for example—-and were quick to enlist the assistance of experts in the various branches of science necessary to manufacture medicines. Thus, scientific and inventive ability, a quality discussed in the chapters by Jim Schmidt and Terry Hambrecht, was especially evident in the army drug-manufacturing facilities.

Moore's reliance on talented botanists, chemists, and pharmacists was only one aspect of an impressive record of Confederate scientific collaboration. Likewise, in Northern hospitals, an expert research team of three military surgeons revolutionized our knowledge of neurology. In his contribution, D. J. Canale describes how "American neurology was cradled and developed in the army during the Civil War" by S. Weir Mitchell and his coworkers George R. Morehouse and W.W. Keen, who took advantage of the unique opportunities that the Civil War afforded for the study of diseases and injuries of the nervous system.

During the Civil War, Mitchell served as a contract army surgeon and persuaded his friend Surgeon General William Hammond to open a center specializing in the treatment of injuries to the nervous system at Turner's Lane Hospital in Philadelphia. There, Mitchell, Keen, and Morehouse performed important clinical research on nerve injuries. Their research culminated in the publication in 1864 of *Gunshot Wounds and Other Injuries of Nerves*, which Canale describes as "one of the acknowledged classics of nineteenth-century American medicine."

Mitchell's postwar writing—drawn from his experiences as a Union surgeon—also made him a famed literary figure, and one of his best-known stories is "The Case of George Dedlow," first published anonymously in *The Atlantic Monthly* in July 1866. It has since become a classic of American literature and medicine. Dr. Canale confirms the conventional wisdom that Mitchell used the fictional story of Dedlow, a quadruple amputee, to introduce the interesting "phantom limb" syndrome—the sensation, after amputation, that the absent part is still present—in a popular magazine before it was widely recognized in the medical literature of the day. Dr. Canale also concludes that Mitchell used the story as vehicle to describe many other important consequences of medical care in the Civil War.

For tens of thousands of veterans, amputation was no fiction. Others continued to bear the pain from wartime wounds for many years, and more still were permanently weakened from the long marches, inadequate diets, or disease. Many veterans—to all appearances healthy on the outside—bore emotional and mental scars every bit as debilitating as their comrades' physical ones. In her contribution, Dr. Andersen describes that, during the Civil War, surgeons were beginning to recognize psychological disorders ("nervous diseases") in soldiers, ranging from simple homesickness to more severe cases categorized as "nostalgia" or "soldier's heart," which were marked by troubled sleep, poor appetite, erratic behavior, and even death.

Unfortunately, as a substance abuse expert with the U. S. Army recently noted, physicians of the time "had primitive notions of mental illness . . . psychiatry and neurology were just being born around this time, and they have changed a lot [since] . . . there was no agreed-upon nomenclature and no precision in diagnoses." In fact, one historian recently suggested that "doctors, sensitive to the demands of masculine dignity, were hard-pressed to come up with 'inoffensive terminology.'"[7]

Certainly, our attitudes about "combat neuroses" have matured over time, and we take for granted that psychiatric casualties are an inevitable feature of warfare. It should be no surprise that Civil War veterans carried their "invisible wounds" into civilian life. Anecdotal evidence of problems in Civil War veterans abounds: divorce, domestic abuse, alcoholism, drug addiction, and more. Still, it was only recently that clinical evidence of "posttraumatic stress disorder" in Civil War veterans was verified by mental health professionals. The publication of that evidence in the February 2006 issue of *Archives of General Psychiatry* received widespread attention, not just in the mental health community but also in the mass media—TV, radio, magazines, and newspapers—from America to Australia.

Dr. Judith [Pizarro] Andersen, the lead author of that landmark report, has contributed a chapter on the mental health of Civil War soldiers and veterans. She draws on both anecdotal and statistical evidence to arrive at some interesting conclusions: Nearly two in five Civil War veterans later developed both mental and physical ailments, and soldiers who enlisted between the ages of nine and seventeen were nearly twice as likely as their older peers to suffer disorders. Furthermore, the percentage of a soldier's company killed—on the battlefield or by disease—was also a significant predictor of later problems, presumably serving as a marker for traumas such as witnessing death, handling dead bodies, and losing comrades. The facts support General William Tecumseh Sherman's oft-quoted aphorism: "There is many a boy here today who looks on war as all glory, but, boys, it is all hell."

As important as asking when the story of Civil War medicine begins is the companion question as to when the story ends. It is too easy—and unsatisfying—to state that the story ends with the surrender at Appomattox, nor do the facts support this view. Harewood Hospital in Washington, D.C., didn't shut its doors until a year later. The compilation of statistics, surgeons' reports, and case studies that culminated in the landmark *Medical and Surgical History of the War of the Rebellion* lasted until the late 1880s. President Abraham Lincoln's declaration that the nation should "care for him who shall have borne the battle" resulted in a strong political lobby on behalf of veterans that crafted and expanded a pension system over the following decades.

The expert and lively contributions to this book demonstrate that the Civil War itself did encompass "years of change and suffering." They also prove that the opportunity to examine the medical aspects of the war still exists to this day: Biographies of men, women, and institutions remain to be studied and written, and archives and primary source material remain unexplored and uninterpreted. Furthermore, this book will expose interested readers and scholars to a significant body of relevant literature and other source material that they may not have considered.

Thankfully, there has been a shift in attitudes among informed Civil War enthusiasts towards that conflict's medical casualties, their caregivers, and the challenges they all faced. Nevertheless, the myths and misinformation that still prevail among the general public indicate that there is still work to be done. We—as contributors to *Years of Change and Suffering: Modern Perspectives on Civil War Medicine*—happily and humbly take up that task.

Notes

1. "Southern 'deputy saw bones'..." in *Burlington Weekly Hawk-Eye*, December 31, 1859, p. 1; "300 ignorant doctors let ..." in *Milwaukee Daily Sentinel*, December 26, 1859, p.1; "intelligent young men ..." in *Lancaster Intelligencer*, December 27, 1859, p.2.

2. "Good News for Richmond ..." as quoted in *Lancaster Intelligencer*, December 27, 1859, p. 2; "absurd and foolish ..." as quoted in the *American Presbyterian*, January 5, 1860, p. 3); "an immense throng of citizens ..." as quoted in *Daily Morning Post*, December 23, 1859, p. 1.

3. *Scientific American*, August 3, 1861, p. 75.

4. "much the more destructive" in J. Theodore Calhoun, "Rough Notes of an Army Surgeon's Experience During the Great Rebellion," *Medical and Surgical Reporter*, IX (1862): 303; Paul J. Dougherty and Herbert C. Eidt, "Wound Ballistics: Minie ball vs. full Metal Jacketed Bullets—A Comparison of Civil War and Spanish-American War Firearms," *Military Medicine*, 174 (2009): 403-407.

5. James M. McPherson, *Battle Cry of Freedom: The Civil War Era* (New York: Oxford University Press, 2003), 486.

6. Ira M. Rutkow, Biographical Introduction, Reprint, Francis P. Porcher, *Resources of the Southern Fields and Forests* (San Francisco: Norman Publishing, 1991), vii.

7. "had primitive notions ..." in Aaron Levin, "Civil War Trauma Led to Combination of Nervous and Physical Disease," *Psychiatric News*, 41 (2006): 2; "doctors, sensitive to the demands ..." in Jennifer Travis, *Wounded Hearts: Masculinity, Law, and Literature in American Culture* (Chapel Hill: University of North Carolina Press, 2005), 31.

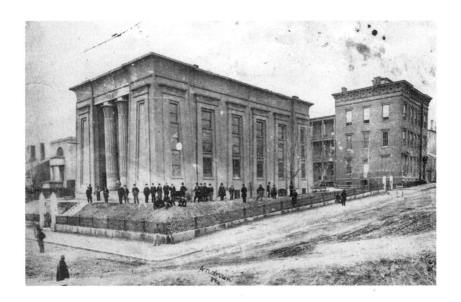

The Medical College of Virginia, as it appeared at the time of the Civil War, consisted of the main college building (foreground), opened in 1844 and designed in the neo-Egyptian style by Thomas Stewart, and the college hospital (far right) completed in April of 1861. *Source: Special Collections and Archives, Tompkins-McCaw Library, Virginia Commonwealth University*

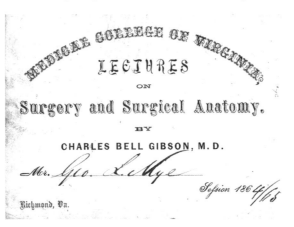

Lecture ticket signed by Professor of Surgery Dr. Charles Bell Gibson authorizing first-year medical student George L. Nye to attend his lectures for the 1864-65 term. *Source: Special Collections and Archives, Tompkins-McCaw Library, Virginia Commonwealth University*

- 1 -

"Medical School for a Nation"
The Medical College of Virginia, 1860-1865

JODI L. KOSTE, M.A.

Secession and war, along with the accompanying turmoil and strife, transformed the largely unheralded Medical College of Virginia (MCV) from a sleepy state institution into the premier medical school for the nascent Confederate nation. MCV's location in the Confederate capital, its stable faculty, and a newly constructed hospital helped to propel the "one horse college" to a place of prominence during the four years of war. A midterm influx of Southern medical students who left their Northern schools in the wake of John Brown's hanging in 1859 fueled the transformation. Enrollment at the Richmond college actually remained high throughout the conflict. This enlarged student body provided the requisite income and critical mass necessary to sustain MCV when other Southern schools were forced to close. The war experience itself gave the faculty chances to provide clinical instruction and undertake new professional activities. These opportunities, combined with the college's commitment to its traditional didactic medical curriculum and anatomical instruction, significantly enhanced the educational experience for matriculating students and helped to catapult MCV to "first in the Confederacy."[1]

Beginnings

The concept of creating a nationally renowned medical school appeared a fanciful dream when Dr. Augustus L. Warner and five other Richmond physicians opened the Medical Department of Hampden-Sydney College on November 5, 1838. The Medical Department operated under the charter of a liberal arts college, but it more closely resembled one of the many proprietary schools that dotted the antebellum landscape. These medical schools existed first for the financial benefit and professional enhancement of the physicians associated with them and secondarily as training centers for aspiring doctors. The Medical Department in Richmond could not count on any endowment or financial support from its parent institution, which was located seventy miles to the west in rural Prince Edward County. Warner and his colleagues began on a modest scale by adapting the old Union Hotel into a medical school building complete with lecture rooms, an anatomy museum, and, most importantly, an infirmary. The faculty promoted the opportunities for clinical instruction extensively, as they attempted to persuade Virginians to stay home for their medical education. Philadelphia's more established schools had long enjoyed the patronage of students from the Old Dominion. While the Medical Department met with modest success in its first decade, it failed to hinder the steady stream of Virginians who headed north for their education or to attract significant numbers of students from neighboring Southern states.[2]

Undaunted by their failure to draw scores of students to the fledgling Medical Department, the faculty spent considerable time expanding the school's facilities. They pushed forward in the 1840s by purchasing land in Academy Square with funds donated by the city of Richmond. A $25,000 loan from Virginia's Literary Fund, secured by a lien on the Medical Department's property, provided funding for a new medical school building. For years the faculty personally bore the responsibility for the six-percent interest payments on the loan. The Medical Department hired Philadelphia architect Thomas S. Stewart to design its new home. Stewart, working closely with Warner, created an Egyptian revival style building, which featured three lecture halls, a top-floor dissecting room, and an enlarged infirmary when it opened in October of 1844.[3]

This modern teaching and clinical building allowed the faculty to expand in additional areas. Following the practice of other schools, the professors created a new chair of physiology and medical jurisprudence in June of 1853 and nominated a physician for the position. The Hampden-Sydney board of trustees selected its own candidate, and a bitter fight erupted. The conflict between board and faculty divided the local medical community and resulted in the dissolution of the Medical Department's connection with Hampden-Sydney. By exercising their political influence and hiring legal advisors, the Richmond physicians secured an independent charter from the General Assembly. The former Medical Department became the Medical College of Virginia in 1854. The new charter did not resolve the school's conflict with a segment of the local professional community, which found an outlet for its censures on the editorial pages of the commonwealth's first medical journal, *The Monthly Stethoscope and Medical Register*. These critics accused the professors of failing to meet contemporary educational standards and of operating the college as a private monopoly for their personal aggrandizement.[4]

The college persevered in the mid-1850s in spite of the acrimonious press war. Detractors accused the college of ignoring the call of the American Medical Association (AMA) for an extended course of medical lectures. The faculty claimed to agree with AMA, but never lengthened the five-month academic year. It did, however, emphasize the importance of bedside instruction as a promotional device and as a means of advocating Southern medical distinctiveness. In response to an AMA survey of medical colleges, the MCV faculty noted that it delivered three clinical lectures weekly and offered, through the college infirmary, "opportunities of observing the diseases of a southern climate at the bedside of a patient, and witnessing the treatment pursued." The theme of a Southern education for those preparing for a practice in the South became a focus as the faculty sought to build the college's enrollment in the years prior to the Civil War. Writing in the college announcement for 1854, Dean David H. Tucker declared, "The Faculty call upon the medical profession of Virginia and the South to second their efforts in behalf of a southern Institution, and give to it that degree of numerical prosperity which is due upon every consideration of self-respect, expediency and patriotism."[5]

Despite Tucker's appeals, MCV remained a provincial school. It enrolled approximately 70 students a term with matriculates primarily from the central and tidewater areas of Virginia. Graduation rates remained stagnant throughout the 1850s as twenty to twenty-six students earned medical diplomas each year. As a point of comparison, the Jefferson Medical College and the University of Pennsylvania experienced record enrollments during this period, with the majority of their students hailing from states south of the Mason-Dixon Line. Jefferson's classes consisted of 500 to 600 students with 175 to 225 earning degrees each year, while the University of Pennsylvania matriculated around 500 students with an average graduating class of 160. Both Philadelphia schools included native Virginians on their faculties and used such men to attract students. Philadelphia-trained physicians in the Old Dominion desired the same education for their sons and apprentices as they had received. They routinely advised potential medical students to head north for their formal education and to bypass the four Virginia medical schools that operated in the early 1850s.[6]

This pattern might have continued indefinitely if not for John Brown's raid on Harper's Ferry and the escalating abolitionist activity in the North. Following Brown's hanging on December 2, 1859, in Charlestown, Virginia, several altercations between abolitionists and Southerners took place in Philadelphia. Medical students participated in the mob activity, and four were ultimately arrested. Two young Virginia physicians, Frances E. Luckett and Hunter Holmes McGuire, who conducted a quiz class for Southern students, concocted a scheme that proved to have far reaching implications. Under their leadership, students from both Jefferson and the University of Pennsylvania organized. These students sent out inquiries to see if they might be admitted to medical schools in the South. Luckett and McGuire followed up by sending dispatches to MCV requesting admittance without payment of the normal professors' lecture fees. McGuire hoped that his direct appeal to his cousin, MCV professor of medicine Dr. David H. Tucker, would elicit a favorable reply. The MCV faculty voted to admit the students on their terms, as did the Medical College of the State of South Carolina.[7]

Led by Lucket and McGuire, the Southern medical students planned a mass exodus from Philadelphia on the evening of December 21. Their decision to secede was dispatched to newspapers across the country. In Richmond, Governor Henry Wise and other citizens with antiabolitionist sentiments received the news with enthusiasm. In no time, funds to defray travel costs were promised or secured from the faculty, the Common Council of the City of Richmond, and local citizens. Two hundred and forty-four students arrived in Richmond on December 22. The students, including over 200 from Jefferson Medical College, the University of Pennsylvania, and other Philadelphia medical colleges, received a hero's welcome complete with a military procession, public speeches, and a grand banquet. The next morning 100 of the original group of 244 continued their journey south. They left behind 144 students who enrolled at the Medical College of Virginia under the liberal terms offered by the faculty. College minutes reveal nothing about the professors' motives in making the generous offer to the students. The faculty may have seen it as a chance to deflect the northern migration of medical students or as an opportunity to expand the alumni base across the South. Whatever the reasons, there is little indication that the professors anticipated how life would change at the college.[8]

MCV became transformed overnight. The provincial school with an overwhelmingly Virginia-based student body now attracted aspiring physicians from as far away as Mississippi and Texas. Some thirty-nine percent of the student body hailed from states other than Virginia, a significant increase over the six percent figure for 1856-1857. Total enrollment for the 1859-1860 session was 228 students, more than two and one half times the previous record high mark reached during the 1850-1851 session. This expanded student body placed MCV in the company of the Medical College of the State of South Carolina, the University of Nashville, and the Medical Department of the University of Louisiana. Each of these institutions regularly enrolled over 200 students in the late 1850s, but these numbers still paled in comparison with those compiled by Jefferson Medical College and the University of Pennsylvania.[9]

At MCV, the increasingly diverse and growing group of students challenged the experienced faculty. They also stimulated the legislature to expand public funding for the college. This public/private partnership would prove critical for the college's survival during the Civil War. One month before the secession of Philadelphia medical students, the MCV faculty laid out plans to seek $5,000 in funding from the legislature to repair and enhance the college's building. By the time the General Assembly considered a bill for support of the medical college, the school's ranks had been swelled by the influx of students. On March 1, 1860, the General Assembly agreed to a generous $30,000 appropriation for construction of a hospital and improvements to the college building. In return, the faculty conveyed its assets, namely the college building, to Virginia's Literary Fund. As the faculty noted in the college announcement of 1860-1861, "the Medical College of Virginia is now not merely under the patronage of the State, but under its absolute ownership and control."[10]

Wartime Faculty

The faculty members who welcomed the seceding students to Richmond would continue to guide the school for the next five years. An examination of their biographical histories offers some insights into the strengths and character of the institution on the eve of the Civil War. The senior member of the faculty was Charles Bell Gibson (1816-1865). He assumed the chair of surgery at the Medical Department following the death of Warner in 1847. Gibson, the son of noted American surgeon William Gibson, studied under his father's tutelage at the University of Pennsylvania, where he earned his degree in 1836. He introduced the use of anesthesia in Virginia and made numerous contributions to the medical literature. One of his former students noted, "He was a very successful teacher, and was indeed the attraction of the College before the war."[11]

For most of Gibson's tenure, David Hunter Tucker (1815-1871) held the chair of theory and practice of medicine. The Winchester, Virginia native received medical degrees from both the University of Virginia and the University of Pennsylvania. After postgraduate training in Paris, Tucker joined several other physicians in organizing the Franklin Medical College. He became the professor of obstetrics and diseases of women at the new school, where he gained a reputation for his lectures. These lectures and his training in Paris formed the basis of his critically received text, *Elements of the Principles and Practice of Midwifery*. In 1849 he was elected to the professorship in Richmond.[12]

The third of the nationally distinguished faculty members, Beverly Randolph Wellford (1797-1870), was a Fredericksburg native and third-generation physician. He earned his degree from the University of Maryland before returning home to practice medicine with his father. In 1852 he served as the president of the Medical Society of Virginia, and a year later he became president of the AMA. He accepted the chair of materia medica and therapeutics at MCV in 1849. Thomas Fanning Wood, a student during the 1862-1863 session who would subsequently serve as a surgeon in the Confederate Navy, recalled that Wellford was "a fine, modest, old gentleman, but a very prosy lecturer."[13]

Four other physicians rounded out the college's faculty. Dr. James Conway (ca. 1820-1865), held the chair of obstetrics and diseases of women and children. He and his colleague, anatomy professor Dr. Arthur E. Peticolas (1824-1868), received their education at the Medical Department of Hampden-Sydney College and returned to the school as members of the faculty in 1856 and 1855 respectively. The professor of chemistry and pharmacy, Dr. James Brown McCaw (1823-1906), joined the faculty just three years before the war. A fourth-generation physician, he studied privately with Valentine Mott and at the Medical Department of the University of the City of New York, where he earned his degree in 1844.

Returning to his hometown of Richmond, McCaw established a practice and subsequently became an editor for the *Virginia Medical and Surgical Journal* in 1854 and the amalgamated *Virginia Medical Journal* in 1856. McCaw's editorial work afforded him an opportunity to collaborate with a number of physicians who would play prominent roles during the Civil War, including George A. Otis and William A. Hammond.[14]

The final member of the faculty was Levin S. Joynes (1819-1881), who served as both professor of the institutes of medicine and medical jurisprudence and dean of the faculty. Joynes, a native of Accomac County, received his A.B. degree from Washington and Jefferson College in Pennsylvania prior to attending medical lectures at the University of Pennsylvania. In 1839 he received his medical degree from the University of Virginia and headed to Europe, where he attended lectures in both Dublin and Paris. Characterized as the most learned man on the faculty, Joynes regularly attended state and national medical meetings and was well known in the profession. After his first year at MCV, he became dean, an administrative position that eventually included a salary. Joynes's leadership, organizational ability, and prudent financial management ensured the survival of the medical college during the four years of war.[15]

MCV's faculty, as these biographical vignettes illustrate, included a mixture of homegrown and Northern-trained physicians. These medical educators brought their new sense of professionalism, their immersion in medical theory and practice, and their international perspectives to bear on the wartime college. Their exposure to broader educational environments in both the United States and Europe prepared them to lead the growing medical school through the dark decade of the 1860s.

Secession

Dean Joynes and the faculty opened the twenty-third annual session on October 1, 1860, six months prior to the commencement of hostilities. Although the faculty was preoccupied with planning for the new hospital and eliminating any deficiency in the educational program, it also confronted another record-size student body. Heightened sectional strife probably stimulated a number of Virginians to seek educational opportunities closer to home. MCV's total enrollment reached 148. Seabrook Jenkins, one of two South Carolinians enrolled that fall, wrote to Dean Joynes in early December requesting permission to sit for his examinations in early January "on the ground of the probable secession of South Carolina from the Union before the end of the present month." The faculty, overrun with similar requests in the preceding term, agreed to Jenkins's petition provided South Carolina seceded before early January.[16]

Requests for early examinations were not the only special accommodations desired by medical students during the 1860-1861 session. R.T. Scott and James M. Park, both of whom matriculated at the National Medical College, in Washington, D.C., sought admission to MCV. They requested the terms that had been offered to the Philadelphia secessionists in 1859. Appealing to the dean's Southern spirit, Scott wrote that "I did not feel willing to be instructed by those who hate myself—hate my home and Institution. I had no other than this motive for leaving the school [National Medical College]. I hope I shall never become so degenerate, so lost to all honor and patriotism, and country pride, as to get my own consent for men who have spent all their lives in assailing the South to instruct me in anything." The faculty members considered the matter but rejected the students' entreaties. Instead they concluded that the professors in question were "not only gentlemen of high professional and personal character, but are entirely free from reproach as to the soundness of their political principles." As the 1861-1862 session began, the faculty learned of another proposed secession by Southern medical students attending Northern schools. The high enrollment of the past term, coupled with the complicated financial accounting that followed the 1859 secession, probably motivated the faculty to offer these students no special terms. Those who desired to return to the South for medical instruction could only enroll and attend lectures after paying the normal matriculation fee and purchasing professors' lecture tickets.[17]

College finances and the secession crisis occupied the thoughts of Joynes and the rest of the faculty in the early months of 1861. Virginia Governor John Letcher called the legislature into session, and by February 4, Virginians were electing delegates to the special convention that would decide the commonwealth's fate. The MCV faculty had already resolved to close the course of lectures as early as February 23 because of the unsettled conditions in Virginia and the country at large. In keeping with past practices, however, the faculty arranged for a graduation supper, planned commencement ceremonies at the Metropolitan Hall, and hired the armory band to celebrate the accomplishments of the 59 young men who passed their final examinations and received medical diplomas on March 1, 1861.[18]

At its first meeting following commencement, the faculty addressed issues related to the nearly completed college hospital. The faculty, hoping to secure an additional appropriation to pay for other college enhancements, invited members of the General Assembly to tour the facility. The Hospital of the Medical College of Virginia, as it was officially designated, opened in April of 1861. The three-story brick hospital, situated on Marshall Street adjacent to the college building, featured eighty beds, gas lights, furnaces for heat, and a large surgical amphitheater, where students could observe operations first-hand. When the hospital opened, the faculty set the same rates it had previously charged patients in the infirmary housed in the main college building. The hospital's opening, however, which might have been considered a purely celebratory occasion under other circumstances, actually occurred under an ominous cloud. The firing on Fort Sumter, President Abraham Lincoln's call for troops, and the Virginia Convention's passage of an ordinance of secession on April 17 would alter the history of the hospital and the college, as well as so many other aspects of Southern life, during the ensuing years.[19]

MCV and the War

The outbreak of war created new challenges for the medical faculty. Professor Charles Bell Gibson assumed a new role as Surgeon General for Virginia. In this capacity, he proposed that the MCV hospital be used for sick and wounded soldiers who could not be accommodated in the various camps around Richmond. The faculty agreed to this arrangement provided that the hospital and the solders admitted to it would remain under its control. Initially, the facility had housed soldiers from Virginia under a contract whereby the state would pay five dollars a week for each hospitalized patient. MCV now negotiated a similar arrangement with the Confederate government. Once the Confederacy institutionalized its medical department, Gibson freed himself to take on other responsibilities. He accepted a commission as surgeon in the Provisional Army of the Confederate States and assumed control of Richmond's General Hospital No. 1 in the former city almshouse, where he had previously presented clinical lectures. The college's location in the Confederate capital allowed Gibson and his colleagues to volunteer for duty with the army while still maintaining their roles at MCV. Other medical schools proved less fortunate. When faculty members from the Medical College of the State of South Carolina, the Medical College of Georgia, and the Alabama Medical College joined the war effort, they were unable to fulfill their teaching obligations in their hometowns. Only four of the fifteen allopathic or regular medical schools in the Confederacy, including MCV, managed to graduate students.[20]

Gibson's colleague, David Tucker, also volunteered for duty and served at Chaffin's Bluff Hospital, General Hospital 21, and Winder Hospital over the course of the conflict. In 1863, he assisted Hunter McGuire in caring for the dying Stonewall Jackson. Tucker and MCV anatomy professor Arthur Peticolas contributed to the Confederate cause by serving on the army medical board. Peticolas collaborated with four other physicians, at the request of Surgeon General Samuel Preston Moore, in compiling a manual of operative surgery, which was published in Richmond in the fall of 1863. Although Beverly Wellford was sixty-four when the war broke out, he offered his services to the military and served in Richmond hospitals. In the spring of 1864, Wellford reported on two different cases of gunshot wounds to the scalp. James McCaw also participated in the war effort. In 1861 Dean Joynes proposed to the surgeon general that he allow the faculty to designate a medical officer for the college hospital who would receive the appointment and pay of a contact physician. McCaw received that appointment but never fulfilled it. He received another commission from Moore to become surgeon in chief of soon-to-be-organized Chimborazo Hospital. James Conway replaced McCaw as the medical officer for the college hospital.[21]

As McCaw prepared for his new role as head of a major military hospital facility, the remainder of the faculty planned for the opening of the 1861-1862 session. The previous June the faculty voted to announce the lectures, having received one hundred dollars each as dividends from the preceding term. Unaware that the other medical schools in the Confederacy would be unable to operate as they had in the past, the faculty aggressively advertised the fall term noting that "the clinical advantages afforded by Richmond during the continuance of the present war, will be invaluable." After two successive terms with a student body in excess of 125, enrollment now fell back to the levels of the 1850s. As Joynes noted in his report to the second auditor's office, the downfall was "a natural result of the disturbed condition of the country, and the derangement of social affairs, consequent upon the outbreak of hostilities, but especially of the active spirit of volunteering, which had drawn into the army, in the first few months of war, the great majority of the young men in the state, and throughout the south." Four Confederate medical schools including the Medical Department of the University of Louisiana, the University of Nashville, Memphis Medical College, and MCV conferred 112 degrees in the spring of 1862. MCV led the group with thirty-five graduates, or thirty-one percent of the whole. The capture of New Orleans and Memphis by Federal forces in the spring of 1862 effectively closed the two medical schools located in those cities. The University of Nashville, on the other hand, continued its educational program in spite of the Union occupation of the Tennessee state capital. Only Nashville and MCV would produce significant numbers of graduates in subsequent years.[22]

MCV's faculty faced numerous challenges while training future physicians during the war. In some ways, the college's fate was similar to other Southern educational institutions. MCV struggled to maintain an appropriate learning environment, obtain supplies, equipment, and textbooks, and remain solvent in the face of exorbitant inflation. Dean Joynes and the other faculty made changes to ensure the continuance of the instructional program. Recognizing that the high cost of living in the Confederate capital presented a hardship for aspiring physicians, the faculty cut the course of lectures from five months to four beginning in the fall of 1862. Students juggled their schedules to fulfill their military responsibilities while simultaneously attending lectures and studying medicine. The faculty members attempted to condense their lectures in order to cover as much course content as possible. Richmond became a hospital center by the fall of 1861, providing many opportunities for clinical instruction. The faculty advised Dean Joynes to confer with the surgeon general about using military patients in the college hospital as subjects of clinical lectures "on the condition of their own consent being first obtained." Students observed soldiers and civilians in the college hospital as part of their clinical instruction. In addition, McCaw took medical students with him when he made rounds at Chimborazo, while Gibson conducted clinical lectures at General Hospital No. 1 to enhance the students' educational experiences.[23]

For almost two years the college hospital admitted soldiers. In 1863, however, the surgeon general required that military personnel be housed in facilities under the control of the Army medical department. During these early war years, the hospital admitted 2,481 patients including 1,861 officers and enlisted men. Escalating prices for provisions, medicine, and other hospital supplies made it difficult for the college to remain solvent. The college attempted to secure fuel and food through the Confederate government. Writing to Inspector of Hospitals Dr. Francis Sorrell, Wellford and Joynes noted, "that the present market prices of provisions and medical stores render it very difficult to fulfil the contract with the Government by which the Hospital agrees to receive sick and wounded soldiers at a certain weekly rate without constant risk of pecuniary loss and embarrassment." Although the surgeon general sympathized with the hospital's predicament, he lacked the authority to order the quartermaster general to provide the needed supplies. When the Confederate medical department stipulated that no more solders would be sent to the college hospital, the faculty decided to discharge the extra attendants, raise fees, and close the wards in the college building.[24]

Dr. W. A. Carrington, Inspector of Hospitals, suggested that the faculty convert the hospital into a facility for officers desiring private care beginning in early 1863. MCV also actively marketed hospital services to the Richmond community. Even with an expanded patient base paying higher rates, the hospital's income could not keep pace with the rising cost of provisions and medicines. Whiskey, a mainstay in the hospital's armamentarium, rose from three dollars a gallon in February 1863 to four in August. Ten months later the college received $90 a gallon for the whiskey it had sold from the hospital's remaining stock. In an effort to offset the high cost, the faculty raised the hospital rates multiple times until February 1864, when it settled on a fee fully seven times higher than the amount charged at the time of the facility's opening. In a last-ditch effort to keep the hospital afloat, Dean Joynes purchased silver and gold coins. He hoped that his hard bullion could buy much-needed hospital supplies from areas outside of Richmond. In the end, no amount of income could keep pace with inflation. As the faculty noted, "the receipts of the Hospital are at present not equal to its expenditures." Raising the rates would reduce even more the number of patients and would offer "no extrication from the present difficulties." The faculty agreed to temporarily transfer the hospital to the Confederate government, but this arrangement could not be negotiated. With no other options available, the faculty members made the painful decision to close the hospital in June of 1864. They transferred the remaining patients to the college building and made the rooms in the hospital available for rent.[25]

War and Administrative Crises

The issues surrounding the operation of the hospital and the college dominated much of faculty's attention during the war years. Accounts management in the Confederate economy constituted a perpetual problem. The professors retained the lecture ticket fees paid directly to them by each student. Matriculation and graduation fees that provided the college's main source of income remained stable until the fall of 1864. MCV initially benefited from the extra income generated by the increased enrollment. Joynes invested it in both Virginia state stock and Confederate bonds, earning $225 in interest between 1862 and 1864. When the cost of supplies and services began to skyrocket as the war entered its second year, Dean Joynes and the faculty found it difficult to match income with expenses. By the fall of 1864, the college had no choice but to raise all of its fees to stay in business. In order to combat rampant inflation, the faculty took the drastic step of doubling student anatomical assessments and graduation charges while quadrupling fees for matriculation and professors' lecture tickets. This income still failed to cover all expenses. Dean Joynes obligated the college to purchase only the bare necessities, which in his mind included the payment of insurance premiums. Joynes understood that the college's two buildings were its only assets, and he faithfully paid for insurance to protect them throughout the war. As late as March 13, 1865, insurance premiums approached $900.[26]

The college's ability to provide anatomical instruction offers a good case study of the way in which personnel instability, rising costs, and procurement problems challenged Dean Joynes and his colleagues. Dr. Marion Howard served as the college's demonstrator of anatomy until his duties as a surgeon in the Provisional Army forced him to leave Richmond. The faculty allowed him to fill his post with a substitute for the 1861-1862 term. Howard resumed his duties as demonstrator while fulfilling his military obligations when he was transferred back to Richmond. The dual job proved difficult. Although corpses remained plentiful in the Confederate capital, finding someone willing to procure and manage them in the dissecting room presented formidable challenges. An exasperated Howard

wrote to Dean Joynes in September of 1863, "The man engaged as a resur-
rectionist [grave robber] is dead; another whom there was some faint hope
of engaging, declines acting, and I am at my wits end for an 'anatomical
purveyor'." On the other hand, the faculty claimed "every facility will be
given for the prosecution of Practical Anatomy, under the guidance of a
competent Demonstrator; and no fears need to be entertained of a deficiency of material for dissection." The cost of providing this educational
experience rose significantly by the third year of the war, and the faculty
implemented a dissection fee at the start of the 1863-1864 term. Shortly
thereafter, Howard resigned as demonstrator. His successor, Dr. Howell
L. Thomas, apparently had greater success in hiring a resurectionist, as
he accepted payments from the college account for anatomical subjects
as late as December of 1864. Anatomical instruction at MCV continued
uninterrupted for the duration of the war and remained an integral part
of each medical student's education.[27]

The war also strained other aspects of the college's life. Beginning in
1862, students had to be concerned about the Confederate conscription act
and the threat of potential legislation that would keep them from attending lectures. The professors also worried about the loss of prospective
students. In the fall of 1862, they asked Dean Joynes to speak with Surgeon
General Moore about exempting matriculating students from the draft. A
year later the faculty petitioned the Virginia General Assembly to extend
exemptions for both medical students and individuals working in hospitals. Students found it difficult to locate the required textbooks because
of the wartime conditions. Ultimately the faculty agreed that students
might use any standard text that could be obtained in the Confederacy.
Reasonable room and board proved almost impossible for students to find
by the second year of the war. The college's location in Richmond also
meant students were potentially in harm's way as the Union Army of the
Potomac directed repeated campaigns to capture the Confederate capital. R. H. Timberlake, a student during the 1864-1865 session, informed
Dean Joynes about potential relocation sites for the medical school should
students and faculty need to flee from an invading army.[28]

Despite these well-documented hardships, MCV continued to function
on many levels. The college always paid and arranged for graduation ceremonies even in the darkest hours of the war. A rite of passage, commencement played a significant role in Southern college life. Traditionally the

faculty hosted a dinner for the graduates following a formal ceremony held in one of Richmond's large assembly halls. The college invited the general public to hear the valedictory address given by a member of the faculty or the board of visitors and to witness the awarding of medical degrees. These practices continued uninterrupted throughout the war in spite of rising inflation, war exigencies, and the military responsibilities of the faculty. Without commencement exercises, the faculty could have no justification for charging a graduation fee, which typically constituted between twenty to forty percent of the college's income. The students also valued these ceremonies. In 1864 and 1865, they donated $185 and $529, respectively, to defray the cost of music at graduation.[29]

The war even provided some unexpected educational opportunities. The Confederate medical department saw that the college could be a valuable training ground for military physicians. Surgeon General Moore devised a program whereby Army hospital stewards with previous medical instruction would be assigned to hospitals in Richmond and granted the privilege of attending lectures at MCV. Following graduation and examination by the Army medical board, they were appointed as assistant surgeons or surgeons. By the end of the war this special consideration was extended to other military personnel who had studied medicine prior to the outbreak of hostilities. Hospital stewards from across the Confederacy contacted Dean Joynes seeking admission to MCV. By late 1864 it appears that many of them were thinking beyond the war and preparing for a future life when they would no longer be in the army. W. A. Hurt, hospital steward in Cahaba, Alabama, who subsequently matriculated in November of 1864, wrote, "The last little wealth that I possessed has just been destroyed by the Yankees in north Miss: and I will have to fall back on my own individual exertions for support after the war. I have shed my blood on more than one battlefield in defense of the liberties we all in common hold dear." Other potential students sought admission following battlefield wounds or worse. Seeking to enroll in the fall of 1864, Edwin N. McAuley informed Joynes apologetically, "I wrote to you last year in regard to attending the Medical College last winter. I was unfortunate enough to be captured while in Penn and was not exchanged in time for the session." Without Joynes's intercession, many hospital stewards would not have secured the requisite transfers or duty assignments to allow them to study medicine. Joynes successfully navigated through the Confederate bureaucracy by meeting with Surgeon General Moore and others in the medical department in order to expedite the application process.[30]

Potential students also appealed to James McCaw for assistance in securing transfers to Chimborazo Hospital, where they might attend the course of lectures at MCV. Some had previously been assigned to the hospital and sought a return to continue medical studies. At times the hospital had more stewards assigned to it than normally allocated, so that these young men could pursue their medical studies while gaining practical experience. McCaw thoroughly understood the Confederate bureaucracy and used it to the advantage of the hospital, the Army medical department, and MCV. He informed the faculty of potential personnel moves that would require some students to abandon their studies when transferred with their military units. In February 1863 he successfully secured his colleagues' approval to hold early examinations for any student who received orders to leave Richmond.[31]

McCaw connected the Confederate medical department and MCV in other ways that directly benefited both the faculty and the army surgeons. He served on the executive committee of the medical department and also participated with several of his colleagues on the various medical examining boards. McCaw's antebellum experience as a journal editor positioned him to have a major role in the production of the *Confederate States Medical and Surgical Journal*, thus creating another professional tie between the medical department and MCV. This publication, conceived by Surgeon General Moore to disseminate information on military medicine to the surgeons in the field, was the only Southern medical periodical to be issued during the war. McCaw, Gibson, and other MCV faculty members made numerous contributions to this journal, which served as the official organ of the Association of the Army and Navy Surgeons of the Confederate States. This association, organized on August 22, 1863, following an invitation from the MCV faculty with an endorsement by the surgeon general, met bimonthly to share case studies, discuss medical topics, and gather data. For its role in organizing the group and providing a meeting venue, the faculty received honorary membership in the association. In return, the professors agreed to host the meetings in the chemical lecture hall of the college building "on the condition of [the association] paying the expenses for fuel and gas." McCaw and Gibson actively participated in the association's meetings, with the former serving as vice president. The last known meeting of the group was set for March 27, 1865.[32]

Two weeks before the last meeting of the Association of Army and Navy Surgeons, MCV graduated its final class of the war years. James McCaw delivered the valedictory address to the sixty-two graduates, who faced an uncertain future. The death of James Conway in February, the closing of the hospital the previous spring, and the liquidation of some of the college's possessions, including the ambulance horse, had cast a pall over the institution. The Board of Visitors planned to meet on April 5 to elect a new professor of obstetrics and to address the affairs of the school. The fall of Richmond however, now altered life in the Confederate capital. As his last administrative act, Dean Joynes paid himself his quarterly salary in worthless Confederate currency. He closed the college's financial books, recording a balance of $1,028.62. In the days that followed, McCaw surrendered Chimborazo Hospital to Union Major General Godfrey Weitzel and his chief medical officer, Dr. Alexander Mott, the son of McCaw's old mentor. Federal troops occupied the college building, which stood in the shadows of the former Confederate executive mansion. During the occupancy, troops destroyed equipment and defaced college records. A final blow came just before the end of April when Charles Bell Gibson, the beloved professor of surgery, died. The remaining five faculty members gathered for the first time following the surrender to eulogize Gibson. They contemplated the challenges that lay ahead for the former medical school of the Confederacy.[33]

Conclusion

In its rise to prominence within the Confederate nation, MCV built an enviable record. Over the course of the war, the college educated 507 students including eighty physicians who returned to the school for an update of their medical knowledge. Almost 200 of the matriculates saw some service time with the Army or Navy. Of the 376 men who received medical degrees from Confederate institutions, MCV awarded 250, or 66% of them. Levin Joynes calculated that seventy-six of the MCV graduates became medical officers. In the MCV catalog for the 1865-1866 session, the professors expressed "much gratification that they have been able to continue their regular course of instruction without interruption during the four years of war with its attendant evils, which have afflicted the country, and they now anticipate the pleasure of welcoming to their halls a large number of young men who have been excluded from them heretofore, by those military exigencies which have opposed an almost insuperable bar to the prosecution of scientific and professional studies." With students and graduates from all corners of the South, a professionally active and engaged faculty, and an educational program supplemented by unique clinical experiences, the college had transcended its provincial roots and established a legacy that would sustain it during the lean and painful years of Reconstruction.[34]

Table 1: Medical College of Virginia, Students by State

State	1856-1857	1857-1858	1858-1859	1859-1860
Alabama	0	1	0	17
Arkansas	0	1	0	4
Florida	0	0	0	0
Georgia	0	0	0	7
Kentucky	0	0	0	0
Louisiana	0	0	0	2
Mississippi	1	0	0	17
Missouri	0	0	0	2
North Carolina	3	5	6	22
South Carolina	0	0	1	14
Tennessee	0	0	1	2
Texas	0	0	0	2
Non-Virginia	4	7	0	89
Virginia	68	53	61	139
Total	72	60	70	228
% Virginia	94%	88%	87%	61%
% Non-Virginia	6%	12%	13%	39%

Table 2: Medical School Matriculates

	1856-57	1857-58	1858-59	1859-60	1860-61
Medical College, South Carolina	234	216	195	196	248
Medical College, Virginia	72	60	70	228	148
Medical Dept of U. of Louisiana	223	258	276	333	402
University of Nashville	n/a	353	436	456	400

Table 3: Allopathic Schools of the Confederacy — Graduates (X = Closed)

	1860-61	1861-62	1862-63	1863-64	1864-65
Alabama Medical College in Mobile	34	X	X	X	X
Atlanta Medical College	60	X	X	X	X
Graefenberg Medical Institute		X	X	X	X
Medical College of Georgia	35	X	X	X	X
Medical College, South Carolina	93	X	X	X	X
Medical College of Virginia	59	35	46	48	62
Memphis Medical College	21	X	X	X	X
New Orleans School of Medicine	76	13	X	X	X
Oglethorpe Medical College	37	X	X	X	X
Savannah Medical College	14		X	X	X
Shelby Medical College		X	X	X	X
University of Louisiana	135	32	X	X	X
University of Nashville	130	22	9	23	21
University of Virginia	10	0	2	1	2
Winchester Medical College	~6	X	X	X	X

Table 4: Weekly Hospital Rates

Date	White Persons, Private Rooms	White Persons, Wards	Slaves and Negroes
Nov. 3, 1860	$7 to $15	$6	$5
Nov. 1862	$15	$10	$8
Jan. 13, 1863	$20	$15	$12
June 1863	$25	$20	$15
Feb. 10, 1864	$49	$56	$35

Abbreviations

TML = Special Collections and Archives, Tompkins McCaw Library, Virginia Commonwealth University

Notes

1. "The Seceding Students" in "Return of the Southern Medical Students Home in 1859," scrapbook of newspaper clippings, Library of the College of Physicians of Philadelphia; John Perkins to "My Dear Doctor" [L. S. Joynes] 15 March 1865, Sanger Historical Files, Special Collections and Archives, Tompkins McCaw Library (TML), Virginia Commonwealth University, Richmond, Virginia. The

institution was frequently called the "Richmond Medical College" or other similar names in the press, in letters, and in other contemporary documentation but this was not the official name for the school.

2. Wyndham B. Blanton, *Medicine in Virginia in the Nineteenth Century* (Richmond: Garrett & Massie, Inc., 1933), 38-49; William F. Norwood, *Medical Education in the United States Before the Civil War* (NY: Arno Press, 1971), 269-72; William G. Rothstein, *American Medical Schools and the Practice of Medicine* (NY: Oxford University Press, 1989), 29-33.

3. The Virginia General Assembly created the Literary Fund in 1810 to provide support for the education of indigent children. It eventually evolved into a fund to support the building and renovation of educational facilities.

4. Blanton, *Medicine in Virginia*, 48-51; *The First 125 Years of the Medical College of Virginia* (Richmond, Va.: Medical College of Virginia, 1963), 14-20.

5. "Medical Colleges of the United States," *Transactions of the American Medical Association* (1848): 293; *Officers of the MCV Session 1853-1854 Announcement of the Session 1854-1855* (Richmond, Va., 1854), 17; John Harley Warner, "A Southern Medical Reform: The Meaning of the Antebellum Argument for Southern Medical Education," *Bulletin of the History of Medicine* 57 (Fall 1983): 364-81; James O. Breeden "States-rights Medicine in the Old South," *Bulletin of the New York Academy of Medicine* 52 (March-April 1976): 348-72. During this period students taking two identical years of courses were eligible to earn their diplomas.

6. Matriculation Book, 1838-1871, TML; Norwood, *Medical Education,* 83; Daniel Kilbride, "Southern Medical Students in Philadelphia, 1800-1861: Science and Sociability in the 'Republic of Medicine,'" *Journal of Southern History* 65 (November 1999): 697-732; "Editorial and Miscellaneous," *Virginia Medical and Surgical Journal* 3 (April 1854): 86-88; Abner Joseph Grigsby to Lucien Grigsby 23 December 1844, Grigsby Family Papers, Virginia Historical Society, Richmond; *Catalogue of the Trustees, Officers, and Students of the University of Pennsylvania Session 1859-1860* (Philadelphia: Collins, Printer, 1860), 11-23; *Catalogue of the Trustees, Professors, and Students of Jefferson Medical College, Session 1859-1860* (Philadelphia: Collins, Printer, 1860), 3-11.

7. James O. Breeden, "Rehearsal for Secession? The Return Home of Southern Medical Students from Philadelphia in 1859," in *His Soul Goes Marching On: Responses to John Brown and the Harpers Ferry Raid*, ed. Paul Finkelman (Charlottesville: University Press of Virginia, 1994), 174-210; Harold J. Abrahams, "Secession from Northern Medical Schools," *Transactions and Studies of the College of Physicians of Philadelphia* 36 (July 1968): 29-45; Minutes of the Board

of Visitors of the Medical College of Virginia 14 March 1860 and Minutes of the Faculty of the Medical College of Virginia 17, 20 December 1859, TML.

8. Breeden, "Rehearsal for Secession," 184-89; Thomas W. Murrell, "The Exodus of Medical Students from Philadelphia, December, 1859" *Bulletin of the Medical College of Virginia* 51 (July 1954): 2-15; and Dean's Report on the Finances of the Medical College of Virginia for the quarter ending March 31, 1860, unpublished report, Sanger Historical Files, TML.

9. See Table 1: Students by State and Table 2: Medical School Matriculates; *Catalogue of the Trustees, Officers, and Students of the University of Pennsylvania Session 1859-1860*, 11-23; and *Catalogue of the Trustees, Professors, and Students of Jefferson Medical College, Session 1859-1860*, 3-11.

10. *Catalogue of the Officers, Students and Graduates of the Medical College of Virginia, Session 1859-60 and Announcement of Session 1860-61* (Richmond: Charles H. Wynne, Printer, 1860), 14; Blanton, *Medicine in Virginia*, 213; Russell V. Bowers, "Civil War Days at the Medical College of Virginia," *The Scarab* 10 (August 1961): 1-3.

11. Donald B. Koonce, ed., *Doctor to the Front: The Recollections of Confederate Surgeon Thomas Fanning Wood, 1861-1865* (Knoxville: University of Tennessee Press), 37-38; Blanton, *Medicine in Virginia*, 55; Howard A. Kelly and Walter L. Burrage, *American Medical Biographies* (Baltimore: The Norman Remington Company, 1920), 436-37.

12. Blanton, *Medicine in Virginia*, 56; Beverly Randolph Tucker, *Tales of the Tuckers: Descendents of the Male Line of St. George Tucker* (Richmond: The Dietz Printing Company, 1941), 26-31; Kelly and Burrage, *American Medical Biographies*, 1164.

13. Koonce, *Doctor to the Front*, 38; Blanton, *Medicine in Virginia*, 55-56; Kelly and Burrage, *American Medical Biographies*, 1280.

14. "Professor James H. Conway," *Confederate States Medical and Surgical Journal* 2 (February 1865): 39; A E. Peticolas to "Gentleman" [Board of Visitors] 10 July 1865, Sanger Historical Files, TML; Blanton, *Medicine in Virginia*, 51, 117; "James Brown McCaw," *Dictionary of American Biography* (New York: Charles Scribner's Sons, 1933), 575-76; and Russell V. Bowers, "Our Faculty in Gray— MCV 1860-1861," *The Scarab* 13 (February 1964): 1-4.

15. Kelly and Burrage, *American Medical Biographies*, 640; Blanton, *Medicine in Virginia*, 50.

16. Minutes of the Faculty 1 December 1860, TML; Matriculation Book, TML.

17. R.T. Scott and J. M. Parks to L. S. Joynes 18 December 1860, TML; Minutes of the Faculty 22 December 1860, TML; R.T. Scott and James M. Parks to "Dean

of the Medical Faculty" [L.S. Joynes] 5 December 1860, Sanger Historical Files, TML; Minutes of the Faculty 17 October 1861, TML.

18. Dean's Account Book, 1856-1871, Sanger Historical Files, TML.

19. Minutes of the Faculty 23 March 1861, TML.

20. See Table 3: Medical Schools of the Confederacy Graduates; Phinizy Spaulding, *The History of the Medical College of Georgia* (Athens: University of Georgia Press, 1987), 72; Joseph I. Waring, *A History of Medicine in South Carolina 1825-1900* (Columbia: South Carolina Medical Association), 84; Rebecca B. Calcutt, *Richmond's Wartime Hospitals* (Gretna, La: Pelican Publishing Company, 2005), 112, 171.

21. The military manual was entitled: *A Manual of Military Surgery* (Richmond: Ayres & Wade, 1863; *The Medical and Surgical History of the Civil War* 12 vols. (Wilmington, N.C.: Broadfoot Publishing Company, 1990), 7: 73, 125, 8: 810; Minutes of the Faculty 5, 12 October 1861, TML.

22. Advertisement for the annual course of lectures, *Richmond Enquirer* 24 August 1861, 3; Report of the Dean of the Faculty of the Medical College of Virginia, 1863, Document 11, Sanger Historical Files, TML; John Duffy, "Sectional Conflict and Medical Education in Louisiana" *Journal of Southern History* 23 (August 1957): 303; Rudolph Matas, *The Rudolph Matas History of Medicine in Louisiana*, ed. John Duffy (Baton Rouge: Louisiana State University Press, 1962, 2:267-68; John Duffy, *Tulane University Medical Center: One Hundred and Fifty Years of Medical Education*, (Baton Rouge: Louisiana State University Press, 1984), 40-41; Philip M. Hamer, "Medical Education," in *The Centennial History of the Tennessee State Medical Association, 1830-1930*, (Nashville: Tennessee State Medical Association, 1930), 365-67. The University of Virginia also remained in operation during the war but graduated only five students.

23. Minutes of the Faculty 29 October 1861, TML; Carol C. Green, *Chimborazo: the Confederacy's Largest Hospital* (Knoxville: University of Tennessee Press, 2004), 110; and Wayne Flynt, "Southern Higher Education and the Civil War," *Civil War History* 14 (June 1968): 211-225.

24. B.R. Wellford and L.S. Joynes to F. Sorrell 5 August 1862, Sanger Historical Files, TML.

25. Minutes of the Faculty 4 June 1864, TML; See Table 4: Weekly Hospital Rates; Minutes of the Faculty 22 May 1864, TML; Report of the Dean of the Faculty of the Medical College of Virginia, 1863, Document 11, TML.

26. Dean's Account Book, Sanger Historical Files, TML.

27. M. Howard to L. S. Joynes 30 September 1863, Sanger Historical Files, TML;

Catalogue of the Medical College of Virginia, Session 1862–1863, (Richmond: Charles H. Wynne, printer, 1863), 12; Marion Howard to the Faculty of the Medical College of Virginia 4 October 1861, TML; M. Howard to L.S. Joynes 22 June 1863, 30 September 1863, Sanger Historical Files, TML.

28. Copy of Memorial to General Assembly 1 October 1863, Sanger Historical Files, TML; R. H. Timberlake to Professor Joynes 21 November 1864, TML; *Catalogue of the Medical College of Virginia, Session 1862–1863,* 15.

29. Robert F. Pace, *Halls of Honor: College Men in the Old South* (Baton Rouge: Louisiana State University Press, 2004), 26; Dean's Account Book, Sanger Historical Files, TML.

30. W. A. Hurt to L. S. Joynes 20 October 1864, Sanger Historical Files, TML; E. N. McAuley to L. S. Joynes 21 July 1864, TML; H. L. Ray to L. S. Joines [sic] 25 September 1864, TML; E. U. Steadman to L. S. Joynes 4 November 1864, TML; J. J. Gravatt to L. S. Joynes 28 December 1864, Sanger Historical Files, TML; Joseph H. McCormick to L. S. Joynes 13 August, 10,14 October 1864, TML.; S. P. Moore, "Address of the President of the Association of Medical Officers of the Confederate States Army and Navy" *Southern Practitioner* 31 (October 1909): 494; H. H. Cunningham *Doctors in Gray: The Confederate Medical Service* (Baton Rouge: Louisiana State University Press, 1958), 36.

31. James L. Hall and James H. Knox to Surgeon McCall [sic] 9 August, 1864, TML; A. L. McCanless to J.B. McCaw 11 October 1864, Sanger Historical Files, TML; Minutes of the Faculty 7 February 1863, TML; Green, *Chimborazo,* 26, 59, 100.

32. Minutes of the Faculty 5 October 1863, TML; Green, *Chimborazo,* 112-14; "Salutatory" and "Association of Army and Navy Surgeons," *Confederates States Medical and Surgical Journal* 1 (January 1864): 13-16; Blanton, *Medicine in Virginia,* 295.

33. Dean's Account Book, Sanger Historical Files; Minutes of the Faculty 4 February, 24 April 1865, TML; Green, *Chimborazo,* 145-46.

34. *Catalogue of the Medical College of Virginia, Session 1863–1864,* 7; John L. Dwyer, "Adult Education in Civil War Richmond January 1861-April 1865" (EdD diss., Virginia Polytechnic Institute and State University, 1997), 126-27; Statement of Graduates 1861-1864, Sanger Historical Files, TML; Matriculation Book; and Report of the Dean of the Faculty of the Medical College of Virginia, 1863, Document 11, TML. Confederate military service derived from unpublished database of Confederate surgeons compiled by F. Terry Hambrecht and Jodi L. Koste.

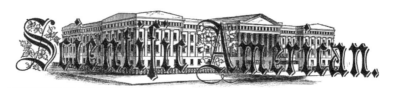

Scientific American.

A WEEKLY JOURNAL OF PRACTICAL INFORMATION IN ART, SCIENCE, MECHANICS, CHEMISTRY AND MANUFACTURES.

VOL. VIII.—NO. 14.
(NEW SERIES.)

[NEW YORK, APRIL 4, 1863.

SINGLE COPIES SIX CENTS.
$3 PER ANNUM—IN ADVANCE.

Improved Projectiles.

When the first note of the present war overspread the land and aroused our people to the necessity of immediate action, it found them utterly unprepared for the struggle. Betrayed on every side, our fate seemed only a swift and speedy destruction. There was scarcely a rifled gun in the country. There were batteries in abundance of the time-honored smooth-bores; there were stacks and mountains, almost, of the bomb-shells and cannon balls which in former days were so serviceable to the nation, but time had rendered these useless. Against iron-clad ships the eleven-inch guns were scarcely better than a pea-shooter against a rhinoceros; and smooth-bored batteries, in action against the long-range rifled guns supplied to the enemy by the English, were of no use at all. In this emergency, what was to be done? America seemed to be in the same condition with Poland, of whom the poet Campbell says:—

"Dropped from her nerveless grasp the shattered spear,
Closed her bright eyes, and curbed her high career."

Our inventors came to the rescue. Like the serpents' teeth sown by Cadmus, which sprang up armed men, the genius and inventive talent of the nation set to work and soon came forward, each one bearing some deadly weapon, or some improved missile, until

at the present time, we fairly bristle with defenses on land and sea. Every town in the land, almost, has its peculiar rifled gun, and shot and shell of the most destructive character can be hurled into the enemy's front, or against his forts, until he gives over the struggle.

The columns of the SCIENTIFIC AMERICAN have contained, from time to time, illustrations and notices of "the grim enginery of war" in the greatest profusion, and the shot and shell herewith illustrated, will convince all intelligent persons that they are of the most formidable kind. These projectiles are those which have obtained a wide celebrity for the inventor, C. W. Stafford. Some of them are very peculiar in shape, and all of them have been proved, by practice, to possess destructive qualities of the highest order. These missiles differ materially from those in ordinary use, and the construction of them exhibits a marked departure from those beaten and well-trodden paths usually traveled by inventors. Although adapted to both smooth and rifled bores, the projectiles have no rifled grooves; they are perfectly cylindrical in shape, being neither hexagonal, nor octagonal, nor of any other form than the one previously mentioned, yet they have, when fired from the gun, as rapid and certain a rotation about

their axis as any rifled projectile. Let us refer to our plate for a description of the individual shot there illustrated.

Fig. 1 is a representation of an incendiary shell, intended for dislodging an enemy from cover, or for burning his towns, ships, barricades, or other defense where he may be hidden. The long wooden case, A, is confined between two metallic caps, B; the shell, C, is cast on the wrought-iron tube, D, and is cored out at regular intervals for the admission of an unextinguishable liquid; this is supplied through the holes, a, now filled by the small screws. The explosive charge is contained in the inner tube, and is fired by a time fuse, E, at the end. The base of the shell is occupied by the metallic plate secured to it by the bolt, b. The recess between the base of the shot and the metallic plate is wound with twine, or any fibrous substance, well lubricated, and the plate itself, at the time of the discharge, is forced into the rifle grooves of the piece, the shell remaining upon the lands; rotary motion is thus imparted, and the missile goes forth upon its errand of destruction and death. Fig. 2 is an elevation of one of these shells with a steel punch head on it.

Figs. 3 and 4 are what are called sub-caliber shot and

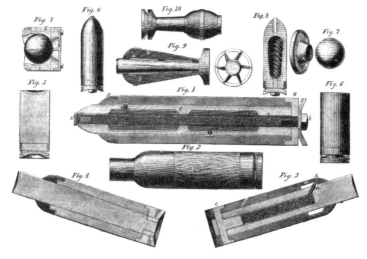

Fig. 7
Fig. 8
Fig. 10
Fig. 8
Fig. 9
Fig. 7
Fig. 5
Fig. 1
Fig. 6
Fig. 2
Fig. 4
Fig. 3

THE CELEBRATED STAFFORD PROJECTILES.

~ 2 ~

"A Multiplicity of Ingenious Articles"
Civil War Medicine and
Scientific American Magazine

JAMES M. SCHMIDT

When viewed through the lens of the American Civil War, George Bernard Shaw's oft-quoted aphorism—"In the arts of life man invents nothing; but in the arts of death he outdoes Nature herself, and produces by chemistry and machinery all the slaughter of plague, pestilence, and famine"—is poetic, but it is also unnecessarily pessimistic. While the inventive genius of the country certainly aroused itself to improving the "arts of death," the "arts of life" were not ignored. The Civil War witnessed innovations in ambulances, surgical implements, medicines, and especially prosthetics.

As America's oldest continuously published magazine, *Scientific American* has delivered opinion and news about developments in technology for more than 150 years. Founded as a weekly broadsheet in 1845 by Rufus Porter, the *Scientific American* of the nineteenth-century was primarily targeted towards inventors and machinists—more like today's *Popular Mechanics* than its own modern counterpart, which expertly reports on the cutting edge of theoretical science. During the Civil War, *Scientific American* played an important role by fostering and reporting on innovations that had an impact on the battlefields and waters.

Scientific American has been used to great effect as a resource in modern studies of mid-nineteenth century military technology. Less attention, however, has been paid to it as a resource in examining patterns of medical-related invention during the era. In fact—just as it did for weapons—*Scientific American* played an equally important role in fostering the arts of life by advising soldiers and their leaders how to maintain the health of the army, urging inventors to give attention to unmet medical needs, and reporting on advances in medical technologies. Study of the magazine's wartime pages also supports recent historical scholarship in the economics and social impact of invention in the nineteenth century.[1]

"The Advocate of Industry and Enterprise"

Born in Boxford, Massachusetts, Rufus Porter was, according to his principal biographer, a "Yankee Da Vinci" with a "grasshopperish interest." With minimal formal schooling, Porter was by turns an apprentice shoemaker, itinerant musician, accomplished painter, schoolmaster, and prolific inventor—his devices included a revolving almanac, fire alarm, washing machine, and revolving rifle—before his interests eventually turned to journalism. In 1840, while living in New York, he bought an interest in a weekly newspaper and soon began a new series of the paper, which he dubbed the *New York Mechanic*. Despite early success for the *Mechanic*, within months, Porter—true to his nature—had found a new interest in electroplating.[2]

In 1845, working as an electroplater in New York, Porter—bitten once again with the publishing bug—invested one hundred dollars to start a new weekly. He called the new journal *Scientific American* with the auspicious subtitle "The Advocate of Industry and Enterprise, and Journal of Mechanical and Other Scientific Improvements." For a subscription fee of two dollars a year, Porter delivered a front-page engraving of an invention (usually his own), news on other recent inventions (often his own), essays on moral subjects, and even some music and poetry.[3]

Despite the originality and breadth of content, Porter's new journal failed to attract a significant audience. The enterprise was also the victim of bad fortune: On October 20, 1845, a fire completely destroyed *Scientific American*'s printing plant, interrupting publication of the journal for three weeks. Porter established a new plant in the Sun building but soon became bored and sold the magazine to Orson Desaix Munn and Alfred Ely Beach.

Munn was born in Monson, Massachusetts, attended school at the Monson Academy, and decided to pursue a career in business. At nineteen, he began work as a clerk in a Springfield bookstore. Two years later, Munn was managing a general store when Beach, a friend and Monson classmate, persuaded him to join in purchasing *Scientific American*. Beach's father was owner of the *New York Sun*, to whose offices Porter had moved his plant after the fire. On July 23, 1846, Munn and Beach bought Porter's interest and his two-hundred-name subscription list for $800.

The men established the firm of Munn & Co. and secured an office in New York City. Munn published *Scientific American* as a periodical chiefly devoted to the interests of the American inventor (discarding Porter's moral essays, music, and poetry) and included a weekly list of all patents issued by the Patent Office. As there was a paucity of expertise in patent law, except in the largest cities, would-be inventors flooded the magazine with requests for advice. To meet the demand, Munn launched the Scientific American Patent Agency in 1847. The agency established a reputation for competence and honesty and became the foremost of its day. In 1860, the agency secured one-third of all patents issued by the U.S. Patent Office.

On the eve of the Civil War, largely due to Munn's direction and head for business, *Scientific American* had become the premier publication of its kind, outliving more than a dozen other technology and science journals launched at mid-century. Porter's quaint four-page broadsheet with only a few hundred subscribers had grown to sixteen pages and boasted a circulation of 30,000.

"Advice to Our Soldiers"

Soon after Lincoln's call for 75,000 volunteers to suppress the Southern rebellion, the Northern press—newspapers, magazines, broadsheets, and journals—carried articles for the benefit of the Union's novice soldiers. Publications large and small—from the *New York Post* to the tiny *Manufacturer and Farmer's Journal* of Pawtucket, Rhode Island—printed letters from Mexican War veterans with practical advice for camp and march, provided suggestions for equipment that should be purchased before mustering in, and even reported on debates over tactics taking place in Rebel circles. The *New York Times* printed a list of "Suggestions from an Old Soldier," whose ten "commandments" ranged from "have plenty of buttons, needle, and thread . . . in your knapsack" to "put a piece of cork . . . in the mouth of your gun to keep out the rain."[4]

One military historian has suggested, though, that of all the contemporary publications, *Scientific American* appeared "to have most consistently served as a means of popular military instruction during the first months of the conflict." The magazine printed articles such as "Learning to Shoot," "Careful Loading of Rifles," and "Disabling Cannon" within the first weeks of the war. The editors also expounded on more esoteric points, such as emerging military theory. In an article entitled "Practical Warfare," the magazine pointed to the "complete revolution" that had occurred in Europe over the past decade, and explained how modern tactics—influenced especially by the increased ranges of new and better firearms—differed from "the olden times."[5]

Still, the *Times*'s "Old Soldier" did not limit himself to purely martial matters; he also had advice to ensure the health of the soldiers. Likewise, in early editorials such as "Diseases of the Camp," *Scientific American* admonished young soldiers and recruits to "never forget that those fatal diseases which attend armies, and make more havoc than the attacks of the enemy, are all preventable," and offered their own commandments, including "proper ventilation, scrupulous personal cleanliness, the wearing of flannel next the skin, the moderate use of fresh vegetables and fruits, especially oranges and lemons; regular rations, and partial or complete abstinence from spirits."[6]

More articles followed, such as "Hints to Volunteers," "Protection to Troops from Sunstroke," "Sanitary Measures for the Soldiers," "Purifying Water for Soldiers," and a nearly page-long article, "The *Scientific American's* Advice to our Soldiers—Malaria and its Remedies." When not addressing the soldiers directly, *Scientific American* lectured the military leadership of the "importance that our valiant troops . . . be thoroughly cared for." Another editorial declared that "the preservation of their [soldiers'] health should be just as carefully guarded to ensure efficiency, as good discipline and a supply of ammunition."[7]

While the magazine admitted that the soldier "must be self-reliant, able to cook, wash, mend, and provide for himself," the editors also declared that it was ultimately the *commanders'* responsibility to guard their soldiers against "privations and fatigue." As an example, they pointed to two regiments that arrived together in the Crimea, camped side-by-side, and were exposed to the "same atmospheric vicissitudes and performed like service." Six months later, one of the units had preserved 2,224 soldiers out of a force of 2,676 men, while the other, with a force of 2,827, had less than half as many left. "Rewards are given to colonels of cavalry in whose squadrons is preserved the greatest number of horses," the magazine extolled, adding advice that "like rewards [should be] bestowed on the colonels whose battalions were distinguished for the healthy condition of the men."[8]

The publishers of *Scientific American* did not just hope that their publication — and advice — would make its way into the hands of soldiers and their leadership; they made sure that it did. "We have been sending several hundred copies of *Scientific American*, for a few weeks past, to the troops in the barracks opposite our office in the Park, and purpose to continue the practice," the editors declared in May 1861, promising also "to forward a number of copies to the several regiments located in Washington, and other portions of our country, every week as a gratuity." The magazine encouraged other publishers to do the same, writing, "After the drill duties of the day are over, the soldiers in camp are not only gratified to have something to read, but are morally and intellectually benefited in so doing."[9]

"The Grim Enginery of War"

It is impossible to separate weaponry — what the editors of *Scientific American* termed "the grim enginery of war" — from medicine in the Civil War, as arms were responsible for hundreds of thousands of deaths and many more thousands of wounds on the battlefields. While the actual number of total patents actually decreased in the first two years of the war before picking back up in 1863 — "Where are the inventors?" *Scientific American* asked in exasperation — there was an early and unmistakable increase in the proportion of inventions in the arts of death. "Our inventors came to the rescue," the magazine declared, "Like the serpents' teeth sown by Cadmus . . . the genius and inventive talent of the nation set to work and soon came forward, each one bearing some deadly weapon, or some improved missile, until at the present time we fairly bristle with defenses on land and sea."[10]

Scientific American featured many of these improved — but conventional — inventions on its front cover, but it was deeper within its pages that some of the "mad" and "unconventional" genius of the nation's inventors was exposed, especially in the weekly column known as "Notes and Queries" in which the editors responded on the feasibility of ideas submitted by readers:

> "N.E.B., of N.H.—The attachment to a projectile of wings to mow down the enemy is a very old thing, and we don't see anything valuable in your application of them."

"M.K., of Ill.—An arrangement of reflectors and lenses which would send a focus of light and heat two or three miles, without diminishing its intensity, so that it would set objects on fire with the same facility as an ordinary sunglass, would be novel."

"A.F.F, of Vt.—The attachment of knives to cannon balls in such manner as to be closed when the ball is placed in the gun, and thrown out when the ball is discharged is a very old idea. We do not know whether such balls have ever been used; we never heard of their use."[11]

Of special note is the emergence of ideas for chemical weapons from the minds of aspiring inventors, many of whom sent their ideas to *Scientific American*. They ranged from a "constant stream of scalding water ... poured into the ranks of the enemy" to ordnance containing cayenne pepper or acids, to chloroform "to send the occupants of a fort to sleep when the shells explode." Doubtless the nation's inventors would have engaged in the technological chess match of threats and countermeasures that marked future conflicts. In defending against chemical warfare, Civil War soldiers might have made use of a growing arsenal of artificial "breathing apparatus," including one model that a historian declared as "superior to the ad hoc emergency masks used by the Allies ... in World War I."[12]

While some of the ideas may seem futuristic and far-fetched—even comical—some, such as using cyanide or arsenic, would certainly have had serious medical consequences if put into play. Civil War surgeons—faced with treating victims of chemical warfare—would have been mostly empty-handed. Wartime advocates and aspiring inventors of these types of weapons "described the toxic effects of the agents fairly accurately," one historian declared but added that "physicians were ill-prepared to treat them effectively." Added to the battlefield casualties would be the inherently dangerous industrial environment—and public health consequences—as laboratories and manufactories engaged in production. Even today—except for antidotes such as nitrites for cyanide poisoning or chelating agents for arsenic poisoning—"treating toxic exposure to most of the agents would consist primarily of supportive care."[13]

"Promoting Health and Comfort"
Still, the genius of the magazine's subscribers was not entirely devoted to

designing implements of death and destruction. As one reader eloquently wrote:

> While many of the inventive minds of our country are devoted to the production of the most effective and destructive weapons . . . others are endeavoring to render the hard and monotonous life of our soldiers as comfortable and pleasant as possible, by furnishing them with a multiplicity of ingenious articles adapted to these purposes. Thus all are exhibiting a desire to add something to the one grand object in view, of restoring unity of States and submission to the laws. In this way those who, for various good reasons, remain at home, contribute their mite in a great many ways.[14]

Scientific American reported with "no small degree of pleasure" that its readers were also devoting their inventive faculty "in promoting the health and comfort of our soldiers and marines." Much had been done "to improve firearms and other implements of war" but also to better "those articles and agencies which tend to promote the health of man, mitigate the privations of war, and render the army and navy more efficient." To spur innovation (and perhaps, its own patent agency business?) the magazine often provided seeds of thought for aspiring inventors.[15]

For example, within weeks of the firing on Fort Sumter, *Scientific American* published a short notice entitled, "Inventions of War Wanted Immediately," with the primary suggestion of a "simple, effective machine for cutting out bandages and making lint for army purposes." Also needed was a "flexible india-rubber tube, fitted with a metallic mouthpiece, with some substance . . . to filter and purify the water," so that soldiers on the march could "slake their thirst with fresh water at every running brook, without the danger of swallowing tadpoles or lizards."[16]

In a November 1861 column entitled "Subjects for Invention," the editors endeavored to suggest "a catalogue of subjects or problems that may, we think, be advantageously conned over with a view to further discovery of improvement." Not surprisingly, many of the suggestions were for military use (an armor clad war vessel, "light of draft, cheap, and quick of construction"; a "pocket telegraph;" armored dress; and a tent "that could be quickly converted into a substantial boat" to carry troops across rivers), but the list also included implements for the surgeon and hospital: a "pulse indicator," which the magazine described as a "small instrument for the sick room, capable of application to the wrist of the patient, to show and record the number of pulse beats," and a "saddle ambulance" for mules or horses that was "capable of ready adjustment so as to remove the wounded from the field of battle."[17]

A similar list a few months later called for more devices still, including a "simple and compact device for stretching and supporting fractured limbs" and surgical instruments, especially an improved implement for "extracting balls from wounds."[18]

There was a special need for improved ambulances, in no small part because a dedicated ambulance corps—vehicle and attendants—was a relatively new development in military history. While hammocks or stretchers borne by horses were used as far back as the Crusades, it was the late eighteenth century before Napoleon Bonaparte's chief physician instituted a "flying ambulance" corps of two- and four-wheeled horse-drawn wagons to remove the wounded from the battlefield. The authors of the official history of medical care in the Civil War noted that vehicles designed as ambulances had not been used in the United States Army until a year or so before the outbreak of the war.

Boards of medical officers considered various models of wagons in the pre-war years, and several designs were used in the first years of the Civil War. Still, they proved unsatisfactory; one soldier, writing of the "privilege" of ambulance transportation, recalled "being violently tossed from side-to-side . . . being tortured, racked, and jolted." The need for an improved ambulance, then, was called for from several corners, including *Scientific American*, which—within weeks of the firing on Fort Sumter—asked that inventors give special attention to "improving the conveyances which serve to carry the wounded from the battlefields," as the wagons then in use were "altogether insufficient in a bloody battle."[19]

When *Scientific American* wasn't suggesting an improved ambulance itself, its attentive readers did instead. R. T. Campbell, writing from Washington, D.C., wrote to "call the attention of inventors to the fact, that we have not a single ambulance in our army . . . deemed suitable for the transportation of the sick and wounded men." Campbell could find only a handful of patents granted for ambulances, found none of them suitable for army use, and was certain that a "really good ambulance would be accepted immediately by our Government, which has shown the greatest liberality to all its soldiers in supplying them with comforts unknown to any European army, and I trust that our inventors will turn their minds in this channel and supply the want."[20]

"*The Arts of Life*"

While the arts of life were undoubtedly outweighed by the arts of death during the American Civil War, there was still considerable activity devoted to improved surgical and dental implements, stretchers, and other devices to aid in camp and in the hospitals, including a "portable mosquito net" (patented through *Scientific American's* agency). Three categories — ambulances, prosthetics, and medicines — received considerable attention from inventors.[21]

Inventors proposed no less than a dozen improved ambulances and scores of improvements in carriage joints, bodies, endgates, frames, dashboards, netting, and medical supply storage, all of which served to improve the mechanics and appliances of the wagons. *Scientific American* was especially enamored with G. W. Arnold's late war invention, with its "novel manner of arranging couches . . . whereby the couches are retained in a proper position when the ambulance is passing over inclined ground . . . being also allowed to yield or give vertically under the jarring movement of the ambulance, and all so arranged as to afford the greatest possible degree of ease and comfort to the wounded."[22]

Prosthetics witnessed a particularly large increase in inventive activity: patents for artificial limbs increased from less than thirty in the previous decade to more than a hundred in the 1860s. "The havoc of war has begotten a multitude of inventions to supply the place of amputated arms and legs," T. C. Theaker, the Commissioner of Patents, wrote in his *Annual Report* of 1865, adding a poignant note of a soldier who "sent a letter to the office written by an artificial arm and hand of his own invention." More than any other medical-related inventive activity during the war, the output of prosthetic designers seems to reflect a response to what they saw as a fruitful market as the government expanded legislation to provide funds for prosthetics to maimed soldiers and sailors.[23]

Theaker, sufficiently impressed at the "high state of improvement" in prosthetics, added that "the United States are in advance of other countries at present in regard to this invention. Some of the legs and arms presented are of beautiful finish and model, and one of the substantial improvements

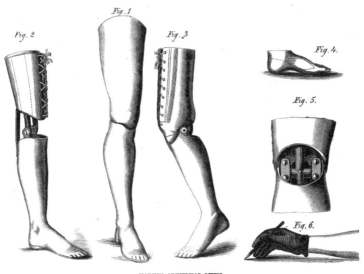

MARKS'S ARTIFICIAL LIMBS.

Engraving of artificial limbs from wartime *Scientific American*

is in the material by which very strong limbs are made with very little weight . . . In one instance the several motions of flexing and extending the arm and fingers has been very successfully accomplished by the several motions that could be made by a stump of the humerus or upper arm."[24]

While admitting that "no art ever shown, if it ever will, can compare with 'nature's handiwork,'" *Scientific American* agreed that the improvements in artificial limbs attained during the war "have caused a great change for the better in the appearance of those who have lost natural limbs, and must give great relief to the maimed." Perhaps it was finish, model, and especially "motion" that so appealed to *Scientific American* such that it often featured new artificial limbs more than any other medical invention during the war in longer articles and elegant engravings, especially when the patents were secured through the magazine's agency.[25]

A variety of nostrums—so-called "patent medicines"—were peddled to soldiers from sutlers' wagons, and with a change to the patent law in 1860, the war generated applications for compounds, oils, ointments, salves, and other remedies. Some of these were designed for the home ("Improved Medicine for Croup" and several "hair restoratives") but many were certainly (even explicitly) for the benefit of the soldiery. For example,

John Weaver's "Improved Medical Compound for the Cure of Diarrhea" was intended as a "speedy and effectual remedy for the disease ... from the attacks of which soldiers in camp are great and frequent sufferers." Others included an "Improved Medical Compound for Miasmatic Diseases," "Improved Composition for Disinfecting and Purifying Hospitals, Camps, and Etc.," and Anson Dart's "Improved Compound Oil" for "protection against ... venereal diseases."[26]

Like many remedies of the era, most of the patented medicines had a vegetable or mineral origin, sometimes of an exotic nature. Dart's preventative was purportedly composed of "an oil of the dwarf olive" and an oil from the seeds of a musk-melon "not known to grow anywhere except in Hindostan." *Scientific American*—with some justification—was dubious of the medicines and remarked on them with bemusement. On the other hand, the magazine reported enthusiastically and presciently on the promise of the emerging age of synthetic chemistry, writing that "Valuable as have been the fruits of chemical inquiry, still more may be expected from the further prosecution of this study," and that the "connection between medicine and chemistry ... will be productive of benefits, the importance of which we can scarcely venture to estimate in the present state of our knowledge."[27]

Especially noteworthy is the fact that women significantly increased their patenting activity during the Civil War. Women accounted for fewer than eighty U. S. patents for all the years up to 1861 but were responsible for nearly ninety patents in the war years alone. To be sure, a good number of these were for household innovations or for items like "Improvements in Corsets," but they also included an "Improved War Vessel" and many medical inventions, including bandages, salves and ointments, and ambulances.[28]

Some inventions by women were explicitly borne of wartime service or perceived needs. For example, in describing the specifications of her "Improved Table for Hospitals," Sarah Hussey made note of her "long experience as a nurse in the United States Army hospitals." Likewise, in describing her "Improved Nitrated Mercurial Ointment," Caroline Learned stated its principal use as "the destruction of vermin which become so exceedingly annoying to soldiers while in the field or camp." One can guess that patents from the immediate post-war period, such as Martha Codman's "Drinking Cup for the Sick" or Lucy Broad's "Improved Disinfectant," also found their genesis in wartime service.[29]

"The Fatal Calamities of War"

War could be a camp-to-grave proposition, and inventors met that grim reaality with more than thirty improvements in coffins, caskets, biers, embalming implements, and Dr. Thomas Holmes's "Improvement in Receptacles for Dead Bodies," a body bag made of India rubber and intended to "facilitate the carrying of badly-wounded dead bodies . . . as the boxes or coffins cannot be so easily handled or transported on the field of battle." In introducing one such innovation, the editors of *Scientific American* solemnly stated, "In the present condition of the country, when the fatal calamities of war render it a duty incumbent on fathers, mothers, wives, sisters and brothers to seek their dead upon the battlefield and to bring home for burial the remains of their kindred, any invention which will tend to ameliorate these afflictions and assist in the performance of this sad duty is worthy of special notice."[30]

In a February 1863 issue, *Scientific American* featured Dr. G. W. Scollay's "Patent Air-Tight Deodorizing Burial Case." The long article outlined—rather graphically—the chemical and biological processes of decomposition, then described Scollay's invention, and concluded with details of a successful experiment conducted by the Sanitary Commission for the Surgeon General. The article also featured an engraving of Scollay's

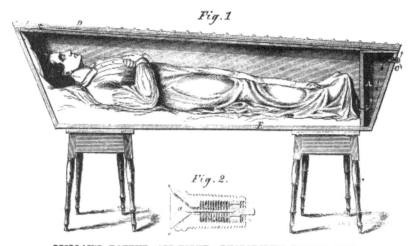

SCOLLAY'S PATENT AIR-TIGHT DEODORIZING BURIAL-CASE.

Engraving of Scollay's "Deodorizing Burial Case" from *Scientific American*

case with a fallen soldier as its occupant. "Especially at the present time is its introduction to be desired," the editors declared, "when desolation and grief exist in almost every home in the land."[31]

Surely Scollay represented the archetypal wartime *Scientific American* inventor. He identified an unmet need, invented a solution, secured a patent (Scollay was actually a prolific inventor, holding several patents related to undertaking), and—most important—profited from a lucrative (if grim) market. *Scientific American* finished its feature on Scollay by directing the "special attention of our readers" to an advertisement for Scollay's invention in the back pages of the issue. "Advertisment" is somewhat of an understatement; it was actually a full column (and then some) of approbation from the Sanitary Commission, Surgeon General William A. Hammond ("I cordially recommend its adoption for army use"), and Valentine Mott, one of America's most esteemed surgeons.[32]

In his endorsement, Mott bemoaned the fact that "in times like the present, when so many are bereft of one or more members of their family by the calamities of a horrid war ....the rich and the titled can afford to be embalmed, but the commoner must be pitched into the pit unheeded and unknown." He praised Scollay's "rare inventive skill" and recommended the burial case to the public so that their loved ones' remains "could be sought and transported to their homes, in order that their bones may rest with their kindred."[33]

The Economics of Innovation

While examining Civil War era medical patents through the pages of *Scientific American* can be interesting, it certainly doesn't tell the entire story; that is, the paucity of medical-related patents (at least in comparison with the "belligerent arts") can give a false impression that there was a lack of medical-related inventive activity. Recent historical inquiry—including evidence from the wartime pages of *Scientific American*—proves the impression false.

This research has centered on the danger of relying solely on patent counts; the revelation that some industries in the nineteenth century had less an inclination to patent than others (a fact which had special consequences for medical invention); the realization that while altruistic inventors are rare, they do exist, and patriotism induced some inventors to freely share their medical-related ideas and devices; and finally, the fact that the immediacy and ethics of battlefield medicine—where necessity truly is the mother of invention—certainly gave rise to *ad hoc* inventive activity.

The fact that patent counts alone are an imperfect measure of inventive activity has been acknowledged by modern economists and social historians; one plainly summarized this truth by declaring, "Not all inventions are patentable, not all inventions are patented and the inventions that are patented differ greatly in 'quality.'" Despite the imperfections, experts in the field have not completely discarded patent records as a measure of inventive activity; some, though, have recently stated that "increasing attention should be paid to the role of invention outside the coverage of patent protection" and that other sources need to be identified.[34]

As an example, one historian specializing in the economics of innovation has made skillful use of data from nineteenth century world's fairs—such as the Crystal Palace World's Fair in 1851 and the Centennial Exhibition in 1876—to examine the direction of invention and the propensity to patent in a nearly a dozen discrete industries. Likewise, a British historian identified the records of the Royal Society of Arts (founded in 1754 as the Royal Society for the Encouragement of Arts, Manufactures and Commerce) as well as the scientific and technical publications of the era—including *Scientific American*—as valuable supplements to eighteenth- and nineteenth-century patent records.[35]

The fair and exhibition data shed light on reasons why medical invention may be especially underrepresented in Civil War-era patents. Fewer than one in five of the more than 7,000 inventors at the Crystal Palace World's Fair of 1851 relied on patents to protect their intellectual property; more important, certain industries were much more likely to seek patent protection than others. For example, the category of "Engines and Carriages" enjoyed a patenting rate of more than 40%, while "Chemicals" and "Scientific Instruments" had among the lowest patenting rates. Perhaps this explains why ambulances enjoyed more patenting activity than medicines or surgical implements during the Civil War.[36]

A sense of patriotism and altruism prompted some inventors to freely share their ideas for the greater good. When R.T. Campbell wrote *Scientific American* of the need for an improved ambulance, he appealed to both the financial and altruistic sensibilities of the readers who might meet the need, adding that the ambulance would "not only be a philanthropic but a remunerative enterprise to the inventor . . . and he will ever afterward have the happy satisfaction of knowing that he contributed some relief to a wounded, or perhaps a dying patient."[37]

Likewise, C. H. Keener, Superintendent of the Maryland Blind Institution, wrote the editors of the *Scientific American* to call their attention to his improvement in stretchers, which he wished to present to the government, "desiring no patent but simply to render to the noble men who may have to suffer on the battle-field this trifling tribute, and I shall feel fully repaid if you deem it worthy of your attention and direct its use wherever requisite." The magazine printed a full description of the novel "pendant stretcher," a handsome engraving, and Keener's declaration that he "did not propose to make them, but to have the Government make them for the army; while I claim no fee for patent or right of invention." The editors complimented Keener on his "sagacity" and on his "patriotism and benevolence toward those men who are suffering all—even death—for their country," and hoped that the stretcher would "be adopted in every hospital and be found on every battlefield."[38]

The immediacy of battlefield medicine also prompted some ad hoc inventions that were never patented or had to wait for perfection. Twenty-five years after the cessation of hostilities, one wartime medical officer still remembered with admiration the ingenuity of his fellow surgeons, writing that when faced with shortages in medicines or other stores, they were "fertile in expedients of every kind." As an example, he recalled an instance when a surgeon broke off "one prong of a common table fork, bend the point of the other prong, and with it elevate the bone in depressed fracture of the skull, and save life." In another, he remembered a surgeon using a "piece of soft pine wood, and bring it out of the wound marked by the leaden ball," before the advent of porcelain-tipped probes.[39]

Finally, professional ethics prevented American doctors from securing patents for medical devices. The American Medical Association (AMA) "Code of Ethics"—first enacted in 1847—proclaimed that it was "derogatory to professional character . . . for a physician to hold a patent for any surgical instrument or medicine" and forbade its members to secure patents. Not all surgeons agreed; Dr. Volney Dorsey—speaking at the Ohio State Medical Society in 1854—declared that "Inventors of valuable instruments are undoubtedly entitled to property and patent rights . . . We should hold inducements to repay them for their expenditure of time, talent, and money, in bringing surgical apparatus to perfection . . . they should suffer no less of professional esteem by endeavoring, in all proper ways to secure it." The AMA did not listen to Dorsey's seemingly reasonable argument and threatened to rescind the Ohio society's membership in the association if they did not toe the line.[40]

Conclusion

Researchers have long used the wartime pages of *Scientific American* as a tool to investigate innovations in nineteenth-century weapons and other military technologies. Less attention has been paid to the magazine as a source for information on medical-related inventions and technologies. The present study demonstrates that while items of the belligerent arts outweighed items of the healing arts in sheer numbers during the Civil War, *Scientific American* also provided advice to soldiers and their leaders meant to ensure and maintain the health of the army, prompted its inventor-readers to give attention to medical-related technologies that would address unmet needs, and reported on improvements in prosthetics, ambulances, medicine, and other inventions. The study also provides an introduction to recent scholarship in the economics and social impact of nineteenth century inventive activity.

In 1862, Henry Adams, son of Abraham Lincoln's minister to England, Charles Francis Adams, wrote his brother in the Union Army, "Some day science may have the existence of mankind in its power, and the human race commit suicide by blowing up the world." Likewise, some time after the Civil War, General Philip Sheridan remarked that the "improvement in the materiel of war was so great that nations could not make war, such would be the destruction of human life." Neither prediction of a world without war or a global suicide has come true, but the acceleration of invention in weapons of mass destruction has. We can only hope that inventors will try to keep pace in the arts of life.[41]

Notes

1. See "The Present Day Use of Nineteenth Century *Scientific American*," in Michael Borut, "The *Scientific American* in Nineteenth Century America," unpublished Ph.D. dissertation (New York: New York University, 1977), 285-88; uses of the *Scientific American* specific to Civil War technology include Robert V. Bruce, *Lincoln and the Tools of War* (Indianapolis: Bobbs-Merrill, 1956) and

Brent Nosworthy, *The Bloody Crucible of Courage: Fighting Methods and Combat Experience of the Civil War* (Berkeley, CA: Carroll & Graf, 2003).

2. J. Lipman, *Rufus Porter: Yankee Pioneer* (New York: C.N. Potter, 1968), 8.

3. For a summary of the historiography of *Scientific American*, see James Schmidt, *Lincoln's Labels: America's Best Known Brands and the Civil War* (Roseville, MN: Edinborough Press, 2008), 185-87.

4. See "The Press as Advisors," Nosworthy, 150-56; "Suggestion from an Old Soldier," in *New York Times*, April 24, 1861, 2.

5. "to have most consistently . . ." in Nosworthy, 151; "Learning to Shoot" and "Careful Loading of Rifles," *Scientific American*, May 11, 1861, 298; "Disabling Cannon," *Scientific American*, June 1, 1861, 340; "Practical Warfare," *Scientific American*, May 11, 1861, 292.

6. *Scientific American*, June 22, 1861, 390.

7. "Hints to Volunteers," *Scientific American*, July 6, 1861, 7; "Protection to Troops from Sunstroke," *Scientific American*, May 25, 1861, 325; "Sanitary Measures for the Soldiers," *Scientific American*, June 1, 1861, 341; "Purifying Water for Soldiers," *Scientific American*, May 11, 1861, 297; "The *Scientific American's* Advice to our Soldiers—Malaria and its Remedies," *Scientific American*, July 20, 1861, 42; "importance that our valiant . . ." in *Scientific American*, May 25, 1861, 325; "the preservation of their . . ." in *Scientific American*, May 11, 1861, 297.

8. "must be self-reliant . . ." in *Scientific American*, May 25, 1861, 325; "privations and fatigue" and others in *Scientific American*, June 29, 1861, 403.

9. *Scientific American*, May 25, 1861, 327.

10. "grim enginery of war" in *Scientific American*, April 4, 1863, 209; "Where are the inventors?" in *Scientific American*, November 22, 1862, 331; "Our inventors came to . . ." in *Scientific American*, April 4, 1863, 209.

11. "The attachment to a . . ." in *Scientific American*, September 7, 1861, 158; "An arrangement of reflectors . . ." in *Scientific American*, September 21, 1861, 190; "The attachment of knives . . ." in *Scientific American*, June 15, 1861, 382.

12. "constant stream of . . ." in *Scientific American*, April 13, 1861, 230; "to send the occupants . . ." in *Scientific American*, June 5, 1861, 382; for an excellent study of the Civil War as a "chemists' war," including many proposals not previously described by historians, see Guy R. Hasegawa, "Proposals for chemical weapons during the American Civil War," *Military Medicine*, 173 (2008): 499-506; "superior to the ad hoc . . ." in Jeffrey K. Smart, "History of Biological and Chemical Warfare: An American Perspective," in Russ Zajtchuk and Ronald F. Bellamy

(eds.), *Medical Aspects of Chemical and Biological Warfare* (Washington, D.C.: Office of the Surgeon General of the Army, 1997), 12.

13. Hasegawa, Proposal, 504.

14. *Scientific American*, December 5, 1863, 358.

15. *Scientific American*, August 17, 1861, 388.

16. *Scientific American*, May 11, 1861, 299.

17. *Scientific American*, November 30, 1861, 346

18. *Scientific American*, March 29, 1862, 204.

19. "being violently tossed . . . " in Reed, William H., *Hospital Life in the Army of the Potomac* (Boston: William V. Spencer, 1866), 57; "improving the conveyances . . ." in *Scientific American*, May 4, 1861, 277.

20. *Scientific American*, December 5, 1863, 358.

21. *Scientific American*, July 23, 1864, 64.

22. *Scientific American*, April 23, 1864, 266.

23. *Annual Report of the Commissioner of Patents for the Year 1865* (Washington: Government Printing Office, 1867), 32-3.

24. Ibid, 33.

25. *Scientific American*, May 13, 1865, 243.

26. "speedy and effectual . . ." in United States Patent No. 41, 3, "Improved Medical Compound for the Cure of Diarrhea," to John Weaver, Knightstown, IN, United States Patent and Trademark Office, Washington, DC (USPTO), January 5, 1864.

27. "an oil of the dwarf . . . " in United States Patent No. 45,028, "Improved Compound Oil," to Anson Dart, Dartford, WI, USPTO, November 15, 1864; "Valuable as have been . . ." in *Scientific American*, August 17, 1861, 99.

28. For an excellent study of female invention in the Civil War era, see Zorina B. Khan, "'Not for Ornament': Patenting Activity by Nineteenth-Century Women Inventors," *Journal of Interdisciplinary History*, 31 (2000): 159-95; for a complete list of inventions patented by females in the Civil War, see *Women Inventors to Whom Patents Have Been Granted by the United States Government*, 1790-1895 (Washington: Government Printing Office, 1895), 4-5.

29. "long experience as a . . ." in United States Patent No. 47,831, "Improved Table for Hospitals," to Sarah J. A. Hussey, Cornwall, NY, USPTO, May 23, 1865; "the destruction of . . ." in United States Patent No. 37,697, "Improved Nitrated Mercurial Ointment," to Caroline Learned, Columbus, OH, USPTO, February 17, 1863.

30. "facilitate the carrying of . . . ." In United States Patent No. 39,291, "Improvement

in Receptacles for Dead Bodies," to Thomas Holmes, Washington, DC, USPTO, July 21, 1863; "In the present condition . . . " in *Scientific American*, February 28, 1863, 136.

31. Ibid
32. Ibid, p. 143.
33. Ibid
34. "not all inventions . . ." in Zvi Griliches "Patent Statistics as Economic Indicators: A Survey," *Journal of Economic Literature*, 28 (1990): 1669; "increasing attention should be . . . " in Christine MacLeod and Allesandro Nuvolari, "Inventive Activities, Patents and Early Industrialization: A Synthesis of Research Issues," Danish Research Institute for Industrial Dynamics (DRUID) Working Paper 06-28, 2006, 21.
35. See Petra Moser, "How Do Patent Laws Influence Innovation? Evidence from 19th-Century World's Fairs," *American Economic Review*, 95 (2005): 1215-1236, and Christine MacLeod, "The Springs of Invention and British Industrialization," *Recent Findings of Research in Economic & Social History*, 20 (1995): 1-4.
36. Moser, 1236.
37. *Scientific American*, December 5, 1863, 358.
38. *Scientific American*, March 28, 1863, 197.
39. H. McGuire, "Annual Address of the President," *Transactions of the Southern Surgical and Gynecological Association*, 2 (1890): 6-7.
40. "derogatory to professional character . . . " in *The American Medical Ethics Revolution: How the AMA's Code of Ethics Has Transformed Physicians' Relationships to Patients, Professionals, and Society* (Baltimore: John Hopkins University Press, 1999), 328; "Inventors of valuable instruments are . . . " G. V. Dorsey, "Report on Surgery," *Transactions of the Ninth Annual Meeting of the Ohio State Medical Society* (Cincinnati: West American Monthly, 1854), 131.
41. "Some day science may . . ." in Chauncey F. Worthington, Charles F. Adams, and H. Adams, *A Cycle of Adams Letters*, 2 vols. (Boston: Houghton Mifflin, 1920), Vol. I, p. 135; "improvements in the . . ." in George S. Boutwell, *Reminiscences of Sixty Years in Public Affairs*, 2 vols. (New York: McClure, Phillips, 1902), Vol. 2, p. 242.

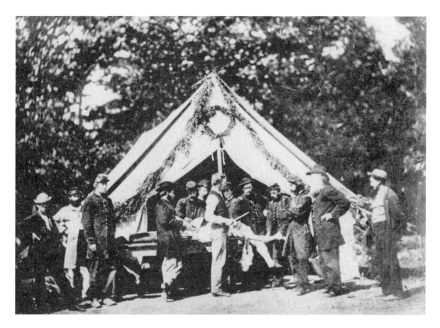

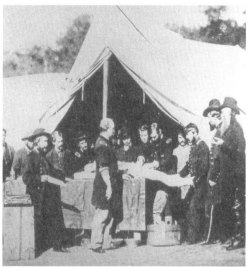

Both illustrations, officially labeled, "Amputation scene at Gettysburg," show a group of consulting surgeons examining a wounded soldier, before making the decision whether an amputation was necessary. *Source: Top photo: National Archives and Records Administration (79-T-2265); Bottom: US Army Military History Institute, Carlisle, Penna.*

~ 3 ~

Amputations in the Civil War

Alfred Jay Bollet, M.D.

At the time of the Civil War, surgery was still rudimentary and the most frequent major operative procedure that could be done successfully was amputation. Many histories of the Civil War condemn the medical care provided during the war, and those criticisms focus primarily on the large number of amputations performed and whether they were necessary. The ill-founded sentiment can be countered if one reviews the nature of the injuries and the medical consequences that led to so many amputations; the reasons, good and bad, for so many amputations being performed; the steps taken, beginning in the second year of the war, to prevent inappropriate amputations; and, finally, the results when compared with other wars of the era.

The assessment of one Civil War historian, Peter J. Parish, that "the medical services represent one of the Civil War's most dismal failures" has been quoted— with and without reservation— in a number of other works ever since. Parish—apparently unimpressed by the momentous advances in medical sciences in the intervening sixty years—emphasized the unfavorable comparisons of the fatality rates of Civil War medicine to the results of the care given during World War I as a basis for the condemnation of Civil War physicians. By the time of "The Great War," medicine had developed the germ theory of disease, identified the organisms that caused the major diseases of the time, including wound infections, and could prevent many of them. For example, typhoid vaccine, available during World War I, almost entirely prevented the disease that killed more Civil War soldiers than any other single disease. X-rays to find bullets and other foreign bodies to aid in their safe removal, major advances in anesthesia late in the nineteenth century, management of fluid balance, and, most important, aseptic surgical technique, had all been developed. But, of course, none of these advances were known to Civil War surgeons.[1]

In making these comparisons, it is worth noting that American military physicians in World War I had a tremendous advantage over their counterparts in earlier conflicts, since Britain had been at war for three and half years before the U.S entered the conflict. In both world wars senior U.S. medical officers—wearing civilian clothes since they were officially neutral—spent several years in England working with the British medical services. When the U.S. entered those wars, senior physicians, with the experience and knowledge gained from the British, became the chief medical officers of the American forces in Europe; in effect, the American medical department entered each war "on the run." That experience, combined with the increases in scientific knowledge and surgical practices, led to the improved results of care of the wounded in "The Great War" and World War II, and—as a case of historical presentism—is not a valid basis for evaluating medical care during the Civil War.

Anesthesia, the greatest advance in medical care of the first half of the nineteenth century, was widely adopted by the time of the Civil War, and was used in almost all the surgery performed; the exceptions were almost entirely limited to instances when supplies had been exhausted. Reports document that raiding Confederate cavalry, when they captured Union supply wagons, made off with as much chloroform as they could carry. For example, on May 24, 1862, when Stonewall Jackson's cavalry captured a Union supply train near Winchester, Virginia, it was the "medical stores," including 1,500 cases of chloroform that they quickly "liberated."[2]

Surgeons performing amputations before anesthesia became available emphasized speed in an attempt to limit the amount of pain inflicted on the patient. By the time of the Civil War, surgical technique had changed little from the preanesthetic days, and the ability to perform speedy amputations, done in only a few minutes, was still considered a desirable attribute of surgeons. The level of anesthesia induced was very light or superficial, further improving safety. Chloroform was the usual anesthetic used in the field during the Civil War, with very few fatalities; since speed was still essential, fatal overdoses of that agent were rarely given. Deaths probably would have been common if the anesthesia was prolonged. Ether, which was safer, was more often used in hospitals.

Before knowledge of bacteriology and the development of preventive measures, infection was a virtually a universal sequel to surgery on any part of the body and in all countries, and infection resulting from opening a body cavity was almost uniformly fatal. Infection of the stump following amputation of a limb led to painful inflammatory swelling (sometimes called "tumefaction") with drainage of foul-smelling pus. Gradually, over weeks to months, this process usually resolved, but sometimes the infection spread and led to fatal "blood poisoning." Infections of amputated stumps, however, healed more often than not.

In contrast, if not amputated, infection of compound fractures (defined as a fracture in which the overlying skin is torn open) almost always led to severe infection that involved the injured bone (known as osteomyelitis). The infected bone and surrounding tissue typically continued to drain foul pus for months to years, often never subsiding completely. Men with compound fractures who were not subjected to amputation frequently remained incapacitated, often bedridden and constantly sick, with recurring drainage of foul pus and fragments of bone from the area. The process could spread unpredictably, leading to "sepsis" or blood poisoning, and death. Most such patients survived the war but died prematurely because of the persistent infection.[3]

Decisions regarding evacuation of wounded soldiers affected the prominence of amputations during the Civil War. Serious head, chest, and abdominal wounds could rarely be treated successfully; as a result of the application of triage principles, extremity injuries were preferentially evacuated to hospitals for surgical treatment, while the more seriously injured were given morphine and not moved unnecessarily. The resulting statistics for the nature of the wounds treated in hospitals has confused students of the war; for example the data in the surgical section of the *Medical and Surgical History of the War of the Rebellion* show that 71% of the wounds were in the extremities, almost equally divided between arms and legs, while only 18% of the wounds were in the trunk and 11% in the head and neck. Military histories of the war have tried to explain these figures, assuming they were totals for all the battle injuries, by suggesting that they resulted from men being ordered to shoot low, and that many arm wounds occurred while men were reloading their weapons. There was only one battle in which all injuries were counted, including those for men "killed in battle." Only 1,173 injuries were counted, but of those killed 51% were in the trunk, 42% in the head and neck, 5% in the legs and 3% in the arms. These data tell us why statistics for hospitalized patients gave the impression that amputations were excessive, since comparatively few other injuries were recorded.[4]

The numbers of killed and wounded were enormous throughout the war, and since about 85% of the wounded evacuated to hospitals survived, large numbers of men with amputations came home and were seen in public after the war. Many families probably had a member who had an amputation. The frequency of amputations and the resulting disfigurement and disability were prominent in the minds of everyone, and that image of the results of Civil War surgical care has dominated the reputation of those surgeons ever since. Indeed, widespread criticism of the surgery performed during the first year of the war appeared in newspaper reports, letters by wounded soldiers, as well as on the floor of Congress.

Medical Director Jonathan Letterman was so disturbed by public criticism of the Army surgeons after the Battle of Antietam in September 1862 that he wrote:

> The surgery of these battlefields has been pronounced [as] butchery. Gross misrepresentations of the conduct of medical officers have been made and scattered broadcast over the country, causing deep and heart rending anxiety to those who had friends or relatives in the Army, who might at any moment require the services of a surgeon. It is not to be supposed that there were no incompetent surgeons in the Army. It is certainly true that there were; but these sweeping denunciations against a class of men who will favorably compare with the military surgeons of any country, because of the incompetency and shortcomings of a few, are wrong, and do injustice to a body of men who have labored faithfully and well.[5]

The wartime criticisms—published and unpublished—affected the judgment of surgeons, making them hesitate to perform amputations even when they were necessary. Instead, attempts were made to save fractured limbs, even compound fractures, without amputation—albeit with some successes—but the resulting infection led to many fatalities or the development of the chronic infections just described.

In deciding whether to amputate, most Civil War surgeons were guided by the aphorism, "every hour the humane operation [of amputation] is delayed diminishes the chance of a favorable issue." (This parallels the modern concept of the "golden hour" for trauma patients).[6]

Late in the war, Dr. Henry S. Hewit, the medical director of Sherman's Army during the 1864 Atlanta campaign, reported, "Secondary and tertiary amputations, after osteomyelitis is kindled or fully established, are very dangerous to life, and every moment of delay in the amputations necessitates a greater sacrifice of length [amputation of more of the extremity]. With a full and careful examination and estimate of contingencies, every case must be decided upon its merits, and it is impossible as yet to promulgate a general law. It must, however, be said that the chances for life, preservation of constitution, and prevention of suffering, preponderate in favor of primary amputation."[7]

William M. Caniff, a visiting British surgeon who was Professor of Surgery at the University of Victoria College in Toronto, visited the Union Army after the Battle of Fredericksburg. He commented that American surgeons were too hesitant about doing amputations: "Although a strong advocate of conservative surgery . . . I became convinced that upon the field amputation was less frequently resorted to than it should be; that while in a few cases the operation was unnecessarily performed, in many cases it was omitted when it afforded the only chance of recovery."[8]

Jonathan Letterman became Medical Director of the Union Army of the Potomac at the end of the Peninsula Campaign, in July 1862. His predecessor, Charles Tripler, had good ideas, such as an organization of an Ambulance Corps, but was frustrated by army regulations designed for the prewar army of about 15,000 men, mostly scattered on frontier posts. Tripler's policy of having regimental hospitals, rather than hospitals serving larger units such as brigades or divisions, was similarly based on prewar considerations and led to a lot of the problems. For example, wounded men had great difficulty finding the correct regimental hospital, often staffed by a single overwhelmed surgeon who had to turn away men from other regiments. Tripler reasoned that the closer the injured man was to his unit, the more likely it was that he would return to duty, but his insistence on regimental hospitals resulted in understaffed units and confusion in arranging care. An even greater problem during that period was the lack of supervision of the regimental surgeons, almost all fresh from civilian life, inexperienced in surgery, and with little knowledge of how to treat severe wounds.

One of the clearest condemnations of army surgeons of the time appeared in the third edition of a standard textbook of surgery used by Confederate surgeons during the second half of the war; it documents that similar problems existed on the Confederate side. Professor J. Julian Chisolm, of Charleston, wrote, "Among a certain class of surgeons . . . amputations have often been performed, when the limbs could have been saved, by inexperienced surgeons, over simple flesh wounds. In the beginning of the war the desire for operating was so great among the large number of medical officers recently from the schools, and who were the first time in a position to indulge this extravagant propensity, that the limbs of soldiers were in as much danger from the ardor of young surgeons as from the missiles of the enemy."[9]

Civil War surgeons, looking back many years later, felt they had performed too few amputations rather than too many. William W. Keen participated in the Civil War as a Union medical cadet before graduating from medical school; after graduation he became an assistant surgeon. Later in the nineteenth century he became Professor of Surgery at Jefferson Medical College in Philadelphia, one of the leaders in American surgery, and a founder of the field of neurosurgery. "The popular opinion that the surgeons did a large amount of unnecessary amputating may have been justified in a few cases," he wrote in 1905, "but taking the army as a whole, I have no hesitation in saying that far more lives were lost from refusal to amputate than by amputating." He added, "Conservative surgery was practiced too much and the knife not used enough."[10]

During the war, the Confederate surgeon and author J. Julian Chisolm expressed concern about the failure to do amputations when needed, and he quoted the official historian of the British forces during the Crimean War, Dr. George MacLeod, who had expressed similar concerns after that war. Discussing this problem, he referred to the difficulty in deciding whether amputation was necessary, and the fear that the British surgeons felt of the criticism directed at them for performing too many such operations. MacLeod, responding to the criticisms that too many amputations had been performed, concluded that "had they [amputations] been more freely practiced [during the Crimean War] . . . a large number of lives would have been saved."[11]

Since the analyses of the Crimean War experience received a great deal of publicity in the late 1850s both in Britain and the U.S., many people in the U.S. were concerned that the same presumed "problem"—too many amputations—which was so widely criticized as a disaster, would also affect American soldiers. These fears only augmented the criticisms of Civil War surgeons starting at the beginning of the war.

On October 30, 1862, about a month after the Battle of Antietam, Jonathan Letterman, after a few months experience serving as Medical Director of the Army of the Potomac, issued an order making a number of administrative changes in the medical department of that army. He changed many of his predecessor's policies, circumventing army regulations (with the approval of General McClellan, commander of the Army of the Potomac). After describing organizational changes such as making the divisional hospital the primary unit, rather than regimental hospitals, the order included the following:

> There will be selected from the division, by the Surgeon-in-chief, under the direction of the Medical Director of the Corps, three Medical officers, who will be operating staff of the hospital, upon whom will rest the immediate responsibility of performing all important operations. In all doubtful cases they will consult together, and a majority of them shall decide upon the expediency and character of the operation. These officers will be selected from the division without regard to rank, but *solely* [emphasis in original] on account of their known prudence, judgment, and skill. The Surgeon-in-chef of the division is enjoined to be especially careful in the selection of the officers, choosing only those who have distinguished themselves for surgical skill, sound judgment, and conscientious regard for the highest interests of the wounded.[12]

It is noteworthy that the selection of the individuals described in this order, as in Letterman's description of his system, was to be based "*solely*" on ability "without regard to rank." The standard army principle of "RHIP," ("Rank Has Its Privileges") was suspended for the duration of the war as far as decisions regarding surgery in the Union Army were concerned.

Later, on May 20, 1864, General Order No. 19 of the Eighteenth Corps of the Army of the Potomac also described the system, stating, "All cases of amputation must either be first designated for operation by the surgeon in charge of the hospital, or be determined upon by a majority vote of a board of at least three surgeons to be detailed by the surgeon in charge, or the corps medical director."[13]

Two wartime photographs, identified as "amputations scenes at Gettysburg," actually show the preliminaries of an amputation. In both, the operating surgeon can be seen standing with his knife or saw ready but not in use. In one of the photographs, another surgeon can be seen standing at the head of the operating table holding an amputation saw. Other surgeons, who will make the decision whether or not amputation is necessary, can be seen examining the patient. These photographs thus illustrate the controls that were established by late 1862, beginning in the Army of the Potomac; they may have been posed because of the long exposure times necessary with the photographic technology of the time, but the scenes seem to depict actual events.

The Confederate army did not have the manpower to copy the system implemented by Dr. Letterman but did essentially the same thing by designating only one surgeon to make the decision while another was given the responsibility to carry out that decision by actually doing the operation. In the third edition of his textbook, Professor Chisolm described the procedure: "In the distribution of labor in the field infirmaries, it was recommended that the surgeon who had the greatest experience, and upon whose judgment the greatest reliance could be placed, should officiate as examiner, and his decision be carried out by those who may possess a greater facility or desire for the operative manual."[14]

During the course of the war a total of 29,980 amputations were reportedly done on Union soldiers with an overall fatality rate of 26.3%. The closer to the trunk the amputation was done, the higher the fatality rate. During the Crimean War fewer amputations were done (a total of 1,177), but the mortality rate was higher at every site (except the forearm and hand) as is shown in the following table:

Fatality Rates After Amputation (%)

	British (Army in Crimea) 1854-56	Confederate (Army of No. Va.) 1861-63	Union (Entire Army) 1861-65
Forearm and Hand	5	12	14
Upper Arm	26	14	24
Shoulder	33	31	. . .

Hip	100	66	88
Thigh	56	38	54
Lower Leg	30	30	38
Foot	23	3	6

Five years after the Civil War, the Franco-Prussian War occurred (1870-1871), and the French were considered the world-leading surgeons at the time. Of the total of 13,173 amputations done on French soldiers during that war, the overall fatality rate was 76%! Although definite conclusions cannot be drawn from these figures, it seems fair to state that, despite the enormous numbers of wounded they had to care for, the results of Civil War surgeons efforts were respectable when compared with international standards of the era.

The negative reputation of Civil War surgeons arose during the war and has changed very little since. Criticisms of the bad practices early in the war were widely publicized, but improvements in care never made it into the newspapers. Because of the huge numbers of casualties in the major battles of the war, many men with amputations, often with artificial limbs (which were made in abundance and included many clever innovations, even functioning replacement arms) were seen on the streets and in homes, but the results of failure to amputate remained unseen, buried.

The experience of one Civil War nurse illustrates the pattern of criticism during the war that was public, but the reevaluation she made later remained unseen in her rarely noted dairy. Mary Phinney, who had married a refugee German nobleman and became the Baroness von Olnhausen, was a widow when the war started and volunteered to become a nurse. It was not until late 1862 that Dorothea Dix called on her and assigned her to a hospital where she was badly treated by the surgeons, who generally rejected Dix's nurses. Phinney's criticisms of the surgeons were copied into many articles on nursing in the Civil War in subsequent years. She persisted despite the maltreatment, however, and soon was accepted and supported by the surgeons. Her abilities became appreciated; she was put in charge of nursing for major portions of the hospital, and the chief surgeon, whom she had disparaged, became a good friend and supporter. She had other major hospital assignments during the war, encountering many other surgeons whom she liked and respected. But after the war ended she felt unfulfilled. When the Franco-Prussian war erupted, she learned German and went to help her deceased husband's countrymen. She summarized her experiences in both wars in her dairy. She wrote, while in Europe, "I feel as if I were back again in our war only here there seems to be no order at all; everyone flies about, distracted. The way they dress wounds is abominable; they are not even where we were in '62.... We never treated amputations so badly.... I can see now how good our surgeons were ..." She added, "How I do long to have one wound in my own hands!"[15]

Mary Phinney later became the first Superintendent of the nursing school established at Massachusetts General Hospital. Her criticisms of the first surgeons she met are widely quoted and are typical of the reputation of Civil War surgery, and the failure of authors to mention her later experiences and overall valuation of Civil War surgery is typical of the literature about Civil War surgery. Despite the evidence that it was better than the contemporary performance of military surgeons in Europe, the quality of Civil War surgery remains underappreciated.

Notes

1. Peter J. Parish, *The American Civil War* (New York: Holmes and Meier, 1975), 147.

2. Robert G. Tanner, *Stonewall in the Valley: Thomas J. "Stonewall" Jackson's Shenandoah Valley Campaign, Spring 1862* (Garden City, NY: Doubleday, 1976), 233.

3. "Sepsis" was a term used by Civil War physicians; it meant a process that included tissue death, resembling the putrefaction of tissue that occurs after death and is derived from the Greek term for putrefaction. The term was often used interchangeably with "blood poisoning."

4. *The Medical and Surgical History of the War of the Rebellion* (Washington, DC: Government Printing Office, 1883), Part 3, Vol. 2, pp. 692, 696.

5. *The War of the Rebellion: A Compilation of the Official Records of the Union and Confederate Armies* (Washington: Government Printing Office, 1870-1901), Series I, Vol. 19, Part I. p. 113.

6. H.D. Riley, Jr., "Confederate Medical Manuals of the Civil War," *J. Med. Assoc. Georgia*, 77 (1988), 104-8.

7. *The War of the Rebellion: A Compilation of the Official Records of the Union and Confederate Armies* (Washington: Government Printing Office, 1870-1901), Series I, Vol. 38, Part 2, p. 524; the terms "secondary" and "tertiary" were used with

varying definitions. In general, "secondary" meant that the initial safe period of a day or two before inflammation appeared had passed, and the amputation was delayed until the swelling and "tumefations" had subsided, usually after a month or two. "Tertiary" amputations were even later after the injury, and frequently were desperate attempts to save the patient months or years later.

8. W. Caniff, "Surgery of the Federal Army (Letter to the Editor), *Lancet*, 1 (1863), 251-2.

9. J. J. Chisolm *A Manual of Military Surgery for Use of the Surgeons in the Confederate Army* (Columbia, SC: Evans and Cogswell, 1864; reprint, Dayton, OH: Morningside Press, 1992), 370.

10. W. W. Keen, "Surgical Reminiscences of the Civil War," *Transactions of the College of Physicians of Philadelphia*, Third Series, 27 (1905), 95-114.

11. G.H.B. MacLeod, *Notes on the Surgery of the War in the Crimea With Remarks on the Treatment of Gunshot Wounds* (Philadelphia: JB Lippincott, 1862).

12. Jonathan Letterman, *Medical Recollections of the Army of the Potomac* (New York: D. Appleton & Co., 1866), 60.

13. *The War of the Rebellion: A Compilation of the Official Records of the Union and Confederate Armies* (Washington: Government Printing Office, 1870-1901), Series I, Vol. 36, Part 3, p. 42.

14. Chisolm, 409.

15. M. P. Olnhausen, *Adventures of an Army Nurse in Two Wars* (Boston: Little Brown, 1903), 231-2.

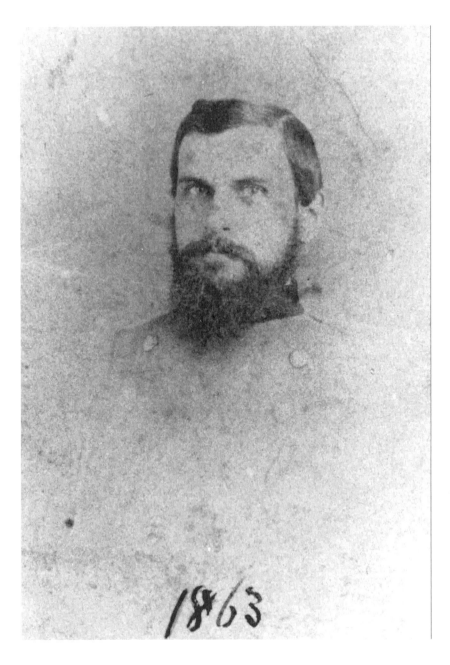

1863

Confederate Surgeon J. J. Chisolm in his uniform
Source: Courtesy of the John J. Chisolm III family; used with permission.

~ 4 ~

J. J. Chisolm, M.D.

Confederate Medical and Surgical Innovator

F. Terry Hambrecht, M.D.

Of all of the physicians who served the Confederacy in a medical capacity, none was more innovative and none, with the possible exception of Surgeon General Samuel Preston Moore, contributed more to the improvement of Confederate medicine than Julian John Chisolm [a.k.a. John Julian Chisolm—see notes]. Most students of Civil War medicine are well aware of his *Manual of Military Surgery,* which was published in three editions during the Civil War, and the pocket-sized anesthesia inhaler that he invented to conserve scarce chloroform and ether. Less well known are his activities as a practicing surgeon during the war, as an organizer of Confederate hospitals, as a designer of a Confederate medical laboratory, and as an improver of medical devices including tourniquets, medical knapsacks, and litters. He also found time to teach his fellow physicians on the proper way to treat sick and wounded soldiers, both medically and surgically.

New information about these activities has been gleaned from the transcription of two letterbooks—one that Chisolm used in Charleston, SC, from November 19, 1861, to June 5, 1862, and the other that he used in Columbia, S.C., from May 24, 1862, to November 14, 1862—and is presented here for the first time.[1]

Before the Civil War

J. J. Chisolm was born in Charleston, South Carolina, on April 16, 1830. He earned his M.D. degree from the Medical College of the State of South Carolina in 1850. Prior to his formal training in medicine, he spent three years in the office of a local practitioner who served as a preceptor. After he received his degree, he continued his studies in Paris. He returned home to practice medicine in Charleston, but again returned to

Europe in 1859. This time he visited military hospitals in Milan where he observed the treatment of wounded soldiers from the Battle of Magenta and the Battle of Solferino in the Second Italian War of Independence. Much of what he learned was used as the basis for his surgical manual. Upon returning to Charleston, he resumed his practice.[2]

In late 1860, Chisolm wrote to then South Carolina Governor William Henry Gist offering his services to the state: "Having had some experience in the recent French campaign in Italy and feeling that I can best serve the state in a professional capacity, by the advice of Gen Wm. E. Martin, I offer my self to you for the position of Surgeon of Brigade, should according to the Military Bill for the defense of the State, a brigade be required for [the] Charleston District." He signed as "Professor of Surgery in the Medical College of South Carolina." This letter is undated, but it must have been written in late 1860 because Gist left office in December of that year.[3]

Chisolm's first medical service in the Civil War was the care he provided to a wounded Federal soldier from Major Robert Anderson's U. S. Army garrison at Fort Sumter in April 1861. An explosion occurred when the Stars and Stripes were being saluted just before Anderson's evacuation. The soldier thought that some of the cartridges prepared for the salute were ignited by the premature explosion of an artillery piece while still within the casemate. He sustained a serious injury to his right eye and his face was "abundantly tattooed by gunpowder marks."[4]

Although Chisolm served in various local units in the Charleston area early in the war, he was not appointed as a surgeon in the Provisional Army of the Confederate States until September 20, 1861.

Hospitals

A hospital known as the South Carolina Hospital was located in Manchester, Virginia, which was directly across the James River from Richmond and connected to it by a bridge. The impetus for the hospital was the South Carolina Hospital Association, which agreed to establish in Richmond, for the accommodation of the sick Carolinians lying at or near that point, a hospital for 150 or 200 patients. The Association agreed to provide the means of fitting it up, furnishing it, and supplying it with all necessary stores, bedding, clothing, food, and so forth. This hospital was organized and opened by Chisolm in early October 1861, making it one of the first general hospitals in the Confederacy. In a letter to Surgeon

Thomas Henry Williams, Medical Inspector of Hospitals for Virginia, Chisolm wrote, "I would state that the South Carolina Hospital will be ready to receive patients on Saturday [October 5] or Monday [October 7] when I will be happy to receive all South Carolinians sick and wounded." An inspection report described the building as a large factory fronting Main Street four stories high with three wards, an apothecary shop, a kitchen, a laundry, a linen room, and quarters for the doctors and a matron. An ambulance and horses were attached to the hospital. By November 8, Chisolm had finished his work in the Richmond area and was back in Charleston, where he signed as "Acting Medical Director."[5]

Chisolm's experience with hospital organization began before the war. In 1857 he had opened a private hospital on Trapmann street in Charleston "exclusively for the accommodation of sick negroes." Shortly after the war began, he offered it to the Soldiers' Relief Association of Charleston. It was accepted and furnished by the association and opened as the Soldiers' Relief Hospital under Dr. William H. Huger. The *Charleston Mercury* extolled in January 1862, "A Committee of Ladies are in daily attendance for the purpose of assisting the officers in their arduous duties, and adding to the comfort and relieving the suffering of the sick soldiers."[6]

In the summer of 1862, South Carolina found itself short of buildings to house sick and wounded soldiers. At the suggestion of Surgeon Robert Alexander Kinloch, Medical Director of the Department of South Carolina, Chisolm contacted the governor of South Carolina about using the buildings of the South Carolina College in Columbia: "As the hospital accommodations in Charleston are nearly exhausted and but small accommodations for the sick and wounded have been elsewhere established, it is desirous of establishing accommodations at once for over 800 sick. It would take months to erect such building. They may be needed tomorrow. The Medical Director desires me to secure from you the immediate use of the College buildings." Six days later Chisolm informed Kinloch, "I have the pleasure to enclose a copy of a letter just received from the Council and Governor of the State tending the use of the entire college buildings [for] the sick and wounded of our army. At the suggestion of Prof La Borde I will visit the buildings tomorrow and see what will be required in the shape of bedding, hospital furniture &c to make the buildings habitable for the sick. The large recitation halls, the two chapels, commons hall &c with the number of small chambers will, I am informed, give accommodation to 3 or 400 sick. I will give you my views after my visit of tomorrow." During the war, Maximillian La Borde was chairman of the Central Association for the Relief of South Carolina Soldiers. After the war, the South Carolina College reopened and he became its president. The college is now the University of South Carolina. [7]

Manual of Military Surgery

During 1861, Chisolm prepared and published the first edition of *A Manual of Military Surgery, for the Use of Surgeons in the Confederate Army*. Noting that no works on military surgery were available in the Southern stores and that the South was experiencing a blockade, he stated in the Preface:

> I saw no better means of showing my willingness to enlist in the cause than by preparing a manual of instruction for use by the army, which might be the means of saving the lives and preventing the mutilation of many friends and countrymen. The present volume contains the fruit of European experience as dearly purchased in recent campaigning. Besides embodying the experience of the masters of military surgery as to the treatment of wounds, I have incorporated chapters upon the food, clothing, and hygiene of the troops; with directions as to how the health of the army is to be preserved, and how an effective strength is to be sustained; also the duties of military surgeons both in the camp and in the field.[8]

Although the number of deaths from disease during the Civil War was twice that from wounds, the ratio was much lower than in earlier conflicts such as the Crimean War, in which the ratio was over six deaths from disease to one from wounds. Since drugs and surgical techniques changed little between these two wars, the application of the principles of public health, as taught in books like Chisolm's, must have been the main contributor to this improvement.

There is evidence that Chisolm's manual was ordered and distributed by the Confederate medical department. In a letter to the Surgeon General, Chisolm asked, "What books shall I issue? I found that my predecessor, Dr. Talley [as a medical director in Charleston] had purchased a number of Chisolm's Manual. Shall the issue be continued?" [9]

Within a year, a second edition was published. After making minor changes, Chisolm delivered the revised edition to the printer, Evans & Cogswell, in Columbia, South Carolina, and told the publisher, West & Johnson in Richmond, Virginia, you have "the exclusive sale of the edition of 1200." [10]

The third and final edition, printed and published by Evans & Cogswell in Charleston, appeared in 1864. Added to this edition were illustrations of surgical operations and some line drawings of medical equipment such as a Confederate field litter and ambulance. Other authors have provided detailed reviews of these manuals, including discussions of Chisolm's thoughts about some of the surgical procedures of the times. [11]

Medical Purveyor, Charleston

On November 19, 1861, Chisolm first signed as "Medical Purveyor, Medical Purveyors Office, Charleston, SC." Before that date, Medical Director R. A. Kinloch had been performing these duties in addition to his responsibilities as a medical director. The principal functions of a medical purveyor included purchasing drugs and medical supplies from sundry sources and distributing them to regiments and hospitals. They were not easy tasks in a nation at war, with little manufacturing capability, and with its ports blockaded by the United States Navy. [12]

As of December 17, 1861, Chisolm was supplying the medical needs of physicians in South Carolina, Georgia, and eastern Florida and receiving many of his supplies from blockade runners coming into Charleston; Savannah, Georgia; and Wilmington, North Carolina. Surgeon William Henry Cumming, the medical director for Georgia, was his contact in Savannah as there was no medical purveyor there at that time. [13]

Having a medical supply depot in the port city of Charleston was precarious because of the danger of Federal invasion from the sea with possible capture of the stores. Chisolm informed Medical Director Cumming in Savannah, "As long as Charleston remains in our possession we will be able to supply you with hospital and medical stores & furniture. Whenever our communication with Georgia is threatened or is cut off I have orders to remove to some central station from which the regular supplies can be drawn. Should necessity require it, it is my present intention to make Augusta that centre." [14]

By May 1862, the danger to Charleston had come to a crisis situation. The

Confederate officer in command of the Department of South Carolina, Georgia, and Florida was General John Clifford Pemberton. General Pemberton advised Chisolm to move inland. In a letter to the Surgeon General, Chisolm outlined his plans: "By the advice of Maj. Gen Pemberton I have commenced to move supplies to Columbia from Charleston. I have not yet secured an office in Columbia and should I not succeed I may be compelled to transfer stores to Augusta. Will you send on the necessary orders to make the transfer from Charleston to the interior to some suitable place for issuing supplies to the army." [15]

Vaccination Against Smallpox

The danger of smallpox was ever present in the Civil War. Forward thinking physicians like Chisolm were thinking of ways of making vaccination more effective. In December 1861, Chisolm wrote to the Confederate Surgeon General, "There has been a demand for vaccine virus and as I understand that it can be obtained in Richmond, I write to you to send me a supply. The *New York Herald's* correspondent from Port Royal speaks of small pox in the Federal Camp. Should it spread among the negros and from them to our troops it will be very destructive. A supply in time may save much trouble." In January 1862, he wrote to fellow surgeon James A. Miller, 18th Regiment, North Carolina Volunteers, at Coosawhatchie, South Carolina, "I also send you a vaccine scab with which you will vaccinate your command." To other physicians in South Carolina, he wrote "I have enclosed some vaccine points which you will use upon your patients," and, "The vaccine points are not very fresh but should only one take, you can from it obtain all the virus you need." [16]

Proposed Designs for Medical Equipment

Chisolm designed new types of medical knapsacks and described them to Surgeon E. W. Johns, who was acting as chief medical purveyor in Richmond: "I am issuing a very convenient hospital knapsack a little larger and twice as deep as the ordinary fare. [It is] divided into 4 compartments surmounted by a horsehair valise. It weighs between 3 & 4 pounds and will carry all articles needed for the battle field. It is much more convenient than the specimen I saw in Richmond and more readily constructed."

In a subsequent letter, he described a field knapsack: "I will send on by tomorrows train a knapsack similar to those which I first issued when leather could be purchased at fair prices but as the exorbitant rates demanded now make the leather knapsack too high for issue I am having them made of duck, not painted, which I think will answer just as well for $7 each. This knapsack will contain everything a surgeon requires on the field."[17]

Chisolm suggested a new field medicine chest to the Surgeon General:

> In issuing medicines to Regiments in the Field there is great waste and destruction of drugs by the difficulty in repacking for the many moves which troops are compelled to make. The small army medicine chest used according to pattern sent from Richmond does not contain 1/10 of the regimental requisition and is a source of general complaint. Would it not be better to issue a chest large enough to contain the entire requisition? If it could be accomplished it would be a great saving in time as well as in medicines. As now arranged requisitions are sent out in large boxes which are unpacked in the open tent and as the articles are in daily use they can not be repacked. They are therefore . . . exposed to theft, abuse, and the destructive influences of the weather. By using large square quart bottles as those at 75 cts per doz in which gin is put up for fluids and tin cans for the powders a very convenient chest can be prepared at a moderate cost.[18]

Written evidence has not been not discovered to prove Chisolm's field medicine chest design was accepted, but a Confederate medicine chest used by Confederate Surgeon B. W. Taylor and presently in the Columbia Relic Room and Military Museum, Columbia, South Carolina, has some of the features he suggested.

Bullet (ball) forceps were used by Civil War physicians to probe bullet wounds and to remove bullets if found. Because there were few surgical instrument-makers in the south, Chisolm relied on a local blacksmith in Charleston to make instruments. In a letter to one of his assistants in Charleston, he suggested a design improvement before submitting an order: "Having had a heavy requisition upon me for ball forceps I wish you would immediately find Mr. Thauss, blacksmith, . . .an order for 100. I had been paying him $3 1/2 for them. Try and have the order filled at $3.00. If he will not reduce the price we must have the forceps. Tell him to make them lighter than the last."[19]

The design of litters, according to Chisolm, left something to be desired.

He shared his idea for improving them with the chief medical purveyor in Richmond: "The two litters which you sent me from Richmond have arrived in good condition. The design of them is not as convenient as those which I am now issuing as the cross bar is liable to be lost from the carelessness of men in camp. I find it more convenient to attach this bar to the side frames by hinges. The hinge costs no more than the iron band and is much more durable." Perhaps Chisolm should have included design changes which made litters more uncomfortable, as he had to complain to the medical director in Charleston "I have understood that General [William Duncan] Smith has reported upon the want of litters among the troops on James Island. These regiments will not have litters when they are wanting as long as the surgeons permit them to be used as beds in express violation of the Med Regulations."[20]

On occasion, Chisolm had to correct design changes in medical devices which were made by others: "I was shown today by Mr. C. Edmondston a tourniquet which you offer as a substitute to those which you have formerly made. Upon examination I do not think that the nail will answer for the buckle and therefore I would not wish you to make any after this manner." [21]

Thoughts on Malingers, Drug Overdosing, and Whiskey

Chisolm often asked the advice of the Surgeon General and was not timid in offering his own thoughts:

> Will you inform me whether the quarterly supply of a regiment is intended to last 3 months. With but few exceptions, notwithstanding the number of sick sent to hospitals, the quarterly supply of leading and expensive drugs is often used out in 3 or 4 weeks and in one instance in a fortnight. What course shall be pursued with such surgeons. Surgeons are apparently not aware of the fact that malingering is very common in the army among many who prefer taking medicine to performing guard duty. Shall I instruct surgeons who I supply, that the quantities put down in the Supply Table for Field Service is sufficient and must hold out the three months. Over dosing is much more injurious than erring upon the other side. [22]

Whiskey was thought to be a medical stimulant in the Civil War era.

Official appointment of J. J. Chisolm as Surgeon, Provisional Army of the
Confederate States
Source: Author's collection

It was used liberally by physicians as an accepted treatment, often to the point of abuse, as illustrated in a letter Chisolm wrote to the Surgeon General,:

> Sir, I would like to have your authority for suppressing a growing evil in the too liberal use of whiskey in the Hospitals. Judging from the large quantity asked for in requisitions it appears to be the common beverage of the sick. Although the requisitions are complied with as to quantity, it is so frequently repeated that I have issued four quarterly requisitions of whiskey in as many weeks. These requisitions have been approved by the Medical Director who does not like to restrict what may be needed. As I can not conceive why whiskey should become the favorite remedy in measles I would ask your authority to limit its use. Patients enter the Hospital sober and leave it drunkards. [23]

Despite Chisolm's misgivings about excessive prescribing of whiskey, he was under pressure to find new sources of it. He wrote to a Colonel J. C. Pickens, Pickens Court House, South Carolina, on May 28, 1862, "Having heard of your reputation as a distiller of good whiskey and being anxious that our sick soldiers should not be poisoned by the vile stuff sold as whiskey, I have written to you to know whether you can furnish any quantity for Government purposes under a State license." As to the quantity needed, Chisolm told a Dr. Moore of Spartanburg, "The government desires to enter into a contract with a good distiller of pure whiskey to furnish 300 bbls at $1.50 per gal." There were problems finding distillers, as Chisolm explained to the chief medical purveyor, "I have corresponded with several parties concerning the distillation of whiskey but have made so far no arrangement. The distilleries in this state [South Carolina] are all broken up and . . . have been sold for the copper." [24]

Solving Problems Faced by Medical Purveyors

When Chisolm became a medical purveyor in Charleston, he was not only responsible for South Carolina, but also for Georgia, eastern Florida, and parts of North Carolina. For the reasons outlined in the following letter, written in February 1862, he urged the Surgeon General to establish additional medical purveyors in Georgia and Florida:

Surgeon Logan who has recently inspected that division of General Lees command located in East Florida complains of utter want of organization in the medical department of that State. They were sadly in want of medical supplies. . . . In Savannah also the organization was by no means as efficient as it ought to be. The Medical Director [in Savannah, GA, William H. Cumming] suggests to me that I should have an agent both in Savannah & Tallahassee. Perhaps you would prefer to establish medical purveyors for both of these cities. As there are but about 4000 Confederate troops in Florida East, and about 10,000 in Georgia (So I am told by Surgeon Logan) ...As the channel of communication may be at any moment cut off from Charleston to Savannah it may be prudent to make some such arrangement as above suggested. [25]

A week later Chisolm recommended to the Surgeon General that a medical purveyor be established in Savannah: "As the Medical Director is still anxious that an agent be sent to Savannah I would recommend for the position Asst Surgeon Wm. H. Prioleau who is familiar with the duties having attended to the duties of the department under Surgeons Talley & Kinloch [in Charleston]." On March 12, 1862, Chisolm informed Medical Director Cumming, "A medical purveyor has been appointed for Georgia. He will be in Savannah on Saturday [March 15]." Chisolm's suggested candidate, William H. Prioleau, was selected. In this new position Prioleau reported to Chisolm, at least initially. Chisolm gave him the following instructions on how to set up his medical purveyors office: "You will find an office and employ an apothecary and porter using all the economy possible $40 for the apothecary and $30 for the porter are the salaries which I am paying and you may employ at the same. You will make inquiry for medical stores such as are issued to the troops and inform me at what prices they may be secured. If supplies can be procured at the same rates as in Charleston the transportation may be saved to the Government. You will make requisition for such supplies as you will require for issue and will in the mean time supply requisitions made upon you through some apothecary in Savannah. You will inquire at what prices store chests, mess chests etc. can be made. The *Medical Regulations* will give you all the general information for your guidance." On March 28, Chisolm sent more instructions: "In supplying requisitions made upon you, you will adhere rigidly to the supply table for field service issuing supplies for one month only and in all instances keeping within the limits there stated. You are ordered also to exercise discretion in making issues and still further curtail those supplies which the character of the sickness among the troops would show not to be required. The great scarcity of drugs and their exorbitant prices should make you exercise every possible economy in their issue."[26]

After moving his main medical purveying depot to Columbia while keeping a smaller depot in Charleston, Chisolm found himself over-loaded. He wrote to Surgeon Johns in Richmond: "From the number of troops which will be kept in Charleston to hold the city . . . would it be efficient to appoint a Field Purveyor for Gen Pemberton? . . . If the suggestion accords with your views I would offer the name of Asst Surg H. B. Horlbeck as an active officer who I think would be well suited for the duties of field purveyor." Dr. Henry Buckingham Horlbeck was an assistant surgeon with the 1st South Carolina Infantry at the time he was selected to be a field purveyor in Charleston. Three days later, after frequent complaints from physicians about the poor service provided by his small depot in Charleston, Chisolm, with the approval of the Surgeon General, closed the depot and ordered most of the remaining supplies shipped to Columbia. However, as he told Horlbeck, he left some items in Charleston for him: "I shall write Mr. Edmondston to turn over to you all the office fixings such as shelving, desks &tc you need or wish, such drugs as you may be willing to receipt for thereby saving transportation, breakage, leakage &c."[27]

When possible new sources of drugs and medical supplies presented themselves, Chisolm did not hesitate to suggest them to the Surgeon General. "An opportunity offers to send to Europe for medical supplies provided the Government will furnish the funds. It would be a savings to the Government of over 100 pc besides obtaining better drugs and in larger quantity. The druggist who proposes going was educated in Germany and is thoroughly conversant with the business. He owns prop-erty in Charleston where he is a native and has his family. I think any funds committed to his care will be judiciously expended and without risk from dishonesty. Will the Government use this opportunity or order as heretofore through Fraser & Co?" Both Chisolm and the Surgeon General

were well aware of the hazards of running the blockade so there was no
need for Chisolm to mention it. [28]

Complaints were lodged against medical purveyors often because of
limitations caused by medical regulations. Chisolm asked the Surgeon
General for guidance on this matter:

> There is a general complaint among hospital surgeons that the supplies
> issued to them from the medical purveyor, in accordance with orders
> from Richmond, are too small in quantity to meet the demands of the
> sick. They ask to be put on the same allowance as for Regiments, viz. 10
> pc or 100 beds to draw the supplies of 1000 men instead of 500. There
> appeared to be reason in their request, as only serious cases are sent to
> the Hospitals, all of which require medicines, and many of which cases
> require their long continued use. They ask for an increase in the staples
> only. How shall I be guided in the issue?

In 1863, the Confederate medical regulation did not change, but
remained as follows: "In General Hospitals, the supplies for every 100 sick
will correspond with the allowance to commands of 500 men. [29]

Administration and Transportation of Medical Supplies

While visiting hospitals in Europe in 1859, Chisolm witnessed the use
of hypodermic syringes, which had been introduced in Europe in 1845.
However, American physicians were slow to recognize their advantages.
In the first edition of his surgical manual Chisolm stated "The endermic [hypodermic] use of this remedy [morphine] would prevent endless
suffering on the battlefield, or in hospital practice." Following his own
suggestion he wrote to Surgeon Johns in Richmond, "Would it not be as
well to introduce the endermic use of morphine as a substitute for chloroform? I think 1/2 gr [grain] introduced under the skin will prepare the
patient in 5 minutes to undergo the most serious operation. I will hunt up
syringes for the purpose."[30]

Confederate medical purveyors relied heavily on railroads for moving
medical supplies. Chisolm devised a rapid and sure method of moving
chloroform from Columbia, South Carolina, to the front in Virginia
when he felt a battle was imminent, as related in a note to his clerk in
Charleston: "100 lbs of chloroform should be carefully packed in valises

and immediately forwarded with all dispatch to Richmond where it has been ordered by telegraph to be at hand for the great battle now hourly expected. The agent who takes charge of the valises should not allow them to leave his presence. They must be taken in the passenger cars with him & he must push on day & night without delay." Unfortunately Chisolm soon ran out of valises, "Valises can not be purchased in Charleston or Columbia. I sent two of my own with chloroform to Richmond and the second agent was compelled to take fifty pounds in a trunk." [31]

Establishment of a Medical Laboratory

Before the end of the Civil War, there were medical laboratories for inspecting and manufacturing drugs in a number of locations in the Confederacy. Before a medical manufacturing facility was established in Columbia, Chisolm took it upon himself to examine drugs and supplies coming into his purveying depot because of problems with substitutions and adulteration. He wrote to a company in Charleston, "I was struck with its peculiar appearance and upon further examining it by the usual tests found that it was not cream [of] tartar at all. I have therefore returned the same." On June 6, 1862, he told a merchant, "The silver [urinary] catheters you have charged at $30 per doz instead of $15 and two of the six are utterly useless, one [is for] a female. The mercury ointment is so weak that the lard is floating in lumps in it. This will also be returned as not in condition to issue to the troops." [32]

In his letters Chisolm revealed some details on the origin of the Columbia laboratory. In a letter to Surgeon Johns, Chisolm suggested, "Would it not be as well to establish a laboratory . . . with the proper appliances which I can obtain in Europe? Arrangements might be made to make & to supply the army during the next campaign or if the Government does not care to embark in this work would it not be an object [of the] to government to invite private enterprise by offering to take . . . men of 65 age to induce the manufacture of such valuable chemicals. Workmen might be obtained from Germany or England familiar with such manufactory." By the fall of 1862, Richmond had approved a laboratory in Columbia, and Chisolm had begun to put it together: "I have prepared a series of copper kettles for boiling the barks for extracts both drug and fluid and have already manufactured some of the barks . . . The tinctures which you have enumerated I will be compelled to make with whiskey as my stock of alcohol is very limited. You speak of one established formula to be used in the manufacture but do not state which. I take the *U.S. Dispensatory* as the standard unless you desire some other formula." The *U.S. Dispensatory* that Chisolm referred to was published in many editions by George B. Wood and Franklin Bache, professors in Philadelphia. The latest edition would have been the 11th published in 1858. [33]

Advising a General

Chisolm grew up in the Charleston area and was well acquainted with the local islands. He wrote to Medical Director R. A. Kinloch, "As you are Genl Pemberton's medical advisor in all sanitary affairs connected with the army, would it not be as well to impress upon him the urgent necessity of making some move or changing the position of our troops, as our stock of quinine is very small, without chances of replenishing it, and that the daily slaughter of our troops by malaria, far exceeds the bloodiest battle we will ever fight there." The Confederates were still on James Island five days later when Chisolm wrote to Surgeon Johns in Richmond, "As the troops situated on the islands in the vicinity of Charleston are in the midst of malaria of the most concentrated character would it not be advisable to issue double supplies of quinine to such troops. In Charleston we have regarded a night spent on these islands during summer months as certain to produce a severe attack of fever often terminating fatally. Hence these lands are shunned after the month of May." Actually Chisolm, with Kinloch's approval, had already begun issuing double rations of quinine to some of the troops "I will issue double supplies of quinine to the most exposed regiments, your approving the requisitions & stating why issued." On June 26, approval was received from Richmond permitting double issue of quinine to all the troops on James Island and other exposed points. Chisolm immediately sent extra quinine from Columbia to Charleston.[34]

After the War

No letterbooks have been found for dates after November 14, 1862. However, isolated pieces of his correspondence indicate that Chisolm remained in Columbia until just before General Sherman led his Federal army through South Carolina. Chisolm was able to escape with some of his stores, first to Chester, South Carolina, and then to Newberry, South Carolina, where he turned what he had over to the Union troops in April

1865. What remained in Columbia appears to have been destroyed, as most of the town was consumed by fire as Sherman's troops were leaving. After the war, Chisolm first practiced surgery in Charleston, South Carolina, and then moved to Baltimore, Maryland, where he became a world renowned ophthalmologist at the University of Maryland. In this position he made original contributions to a medical specialty in its infancy. He died November 1, 1903, in Petersburg, Virginia, after an incapacitating stroke.[35]

Conclusion

The Confederate States of America was faced with many problems, not the least of which was the establishment of a new medical department to care for its sick and wounded soldiers. A few men rose to leadership roles in this department because of their experience, industry, and creativity. Dr. John Julian Chisolm had all of these attributes. He excelled in innovative ideas, many of which were put into practice in the Confederate Medical Department.

Abbreviations

JJC: John Julian Chisolm

SPM: Samuel Preston Moore, Surgeon General, Confederate States Army

EWJ: Edward W. Johns, Chief Medical Purveyor, Richmond, Virginia.

RAK: Robert A. Kinloch, Medical Director, Department of South Carolina

NARA: National Archives and Records Administration, Washington, D.C.

LB-Char: *Letter Book of the Medical Director's Office*, Charleston, SC, Oct. 8, 1861, to Nov. 18, 1861, and the Medical Purveyor's Office, Charleston, SC, Nov. 19, 1861, to June 5, 1862. Entries by Confederate Surgeons A.N. Talley, R.A. Kinloch, and J.J. Chisolm. Transcribed by F. Terry Hambrecht. Author's collection.

LB-Col: *Letter Book of Dr. J. J. Chisolm, Medical Purveyor, C.S.A.*, Columbia, S.C., May 24 to November 14, 1862. Transcribed by F. Terry Hambrecht. Wessels Library, Newberry College, Newberry, S.C.

Notes

Dr. Chisolm signed his name "J J Chisolm." He was christened John Julian Chisolm, and his name is listed as J. Julian Chisolm on all three Civil War editions of his surgical manual. However, on his publications after the Civil War, he preferred the reverse order of names, Julian John Chisolm. His gravestone bears the name J. Julian Chisolm.

1. F. Terry Hambrecht, Michael Rhode, and Alan Hawk, "Dr. Chisolm's Inhaler: A Rare Confederate Medical Invention," *The Journal of the South Carolina Medical Association*, 87 (May 1991): 277-280; Letter book of the Medical Director's Office, Charleston, SC, Oct 8, 1861 to Nov 18, 1861 and the Medical Purveyor's Office, Charleston, SC, Nov 19, 1861 to June 5, 1862. Entries by Confederate surgeons A.N. Talley, R.A. Kinloch, and J.J. Chisolm. Transcribed by F. Terry Hambrecht. Author's collection, LB-Char; Letter book of Dr. J. J. Chisolm, Medical Purveyor, C.S.A., Columbia, S.C., May 24 to November 14, 1862. Entries by Confederate surgeon J. J. Chisolm. Transcribed by F. Terry Hambrecht. Wessels Library, Newberry College, Newberry, S.C, LB-Col.

2. F. Terry Hambrecht, "Julian John Chisolm," *American National Biography* (New York: Oxford Press: 1998), 823-824.

3. Surgeon J. J. Chisolm, Compiled Service Record filed under General & Staff, microfilm M331, NARA; William Henry Gist, *The National Cyclopedia of American Biography* (New York: James T. White & Co, 1906), Vol. 12, p. 172.

4. *Charleston Mercury*, April 22, 1861.

5. *Charleston Mercury*, September 25, 1861; Surgeon J.J. Chisolm, Compiled Service Record; W. A. Carrington, Surg & Inspr of Hosps to E.J. Gaillard, Medical Director, December 8, 1862, Record Group 109, Chapter 6, Volume 416, NARA; JJC to unknown address requesting wire splints, November 8, 1861, LB-Char. At this time, Chisolm was serving as the Acting Medical Director, Department of South Carolina.

6. *Charleston Medical Journal* 12, (1857): 134; *Charleston Mercury*, January 30, 1862.

7. JJC to Governor Francis Pickens, 12 June, 1862, LB-Col; JJC to Surgeon R. A. Kinloch, 18 Jun. 1862, LB-Col.

8. J.J. Chisolm, *A Manual of Military Surgery for the Use of Surgeons in the Confederate States Army* (Richmond, West and Johnson, 1861); Louis C. Duncan, *The Medical Department of the United States Army in the Civil War* (n.p., n.d.); Seaman Prize Essay—The Comparative Mortality of Disease and Battle Casualties in the Historic Wars of the World (n.p, n.d., approx 1910), 20-28.

9. JJC to SPM, 28 Dec. 1861, LB-Char. Dr. Alexander Nicholas Talley served as a medical director in Charleston, South Carolina, in 1861.

10. J.J. Chisolm, *A Manual of Military Surgery for the Use of Surgeons in the Confederate States Army* (Richmond, West and Johnson, 1862); JJC to West & Johnson, 12 Feb. 1862, LB-Char.

11. Chisolm, J. J. *A Manual of Military Surgery for the Use of Surgeons in the Confederate States Army* (Columbia, South Carolina, Evans and Cogswell, 1864);

R. Sherman, "Julian John Chisolm, M.D.: President's Address," *The American Surgeon*, 55 (January 1986) 1-8; H. D. Riley, "Confederate Medical Manuals of the Civil War," *J Med Assoc Ga*, 77 (February 1988): 104-8.

12. JJC to RAK, 19 Nov. 1861, LB-Char.

13. JJC to SPM, 17 Dec. 1861, LB-Char.

14. JJC to Medical Director William Henry Cumming, 2 Dec. 1861, LB-Char.

15. JJC to SPM, 5 Dec. 1862, LB-Char.

16. JJC to SPM, 31 Dec. 1861, LB-Char; JJC to Surgeon James A. Miller, 6 Jan. 1862, LB-Char; JJC to Asst. Surgeon J. J. Jenkins, 6 Jan. 1862, LB-Char; JJC to Surgeon Henry R. Noel, 24 Jan. 1862. LB-Char. Although Civil War physicians did not use the term *virus* in the sense that it is used today, i.e., an ultramicroscopic infectious agent, they were aware that there was something in the discharge that oozed from a successful vaccination that could be used to vaccinate others. They called the active substance *virus*.

17. JJC to EWJ, 17 Dec. 1861; JJC to EWJ, 23 Dec. 1861.

18. JJC to SPM, 16 Jan. 1862, LB-Char.

19. JJC to Asst. Surgeon H. B. Horlbeck, 23 Jun. 1862, LB-Col.

20. JJC to EWJ, 23 Jan. 1862, LB-Char; JJC to RAK, 30 Jun. 1862, LB-Col.

21. JJC to Mr. A. McKensie, 5, Jul. 1862, LB-Col.

22. JJC to SPM, 15 Feb. 1862, LB-Char.

23. JJC to SPM, 26 Feb. 1862, LB-Char.

24. JJC to Col J. C. Pickens, 28 May 1862, LB-Col; JJC to Dr. Moore, 27 May 1862, LB-Col; JJC to EWJ, 7 Jun. 1862, LB-Col.

25. Guy R. Hasegawa, "Confederate Medical Purveying in Savannah and Macon", presentation at the Thirteenth Annual Conference on Civil War Medicine, Hagerstown, MD, 10 Oct 2005; JJC to SPM, 28 Feb. 1862, LB-Char.

26. JJC to SPM, 05 Mar. 1862, LB-Char; JJC to William H. Cumming, 12 Mar. 1862, LB-Char; JJC to William H. Prioleau, 25 Mar. 1862, LB-Char; JJC to William H. Prioleau, 28 Mar. 1862, LB-Char.

27. JJC to EWJ, 7 Jun. 1862, LB-Col; JJC to Charles Edmondston, 10 Jun. 1862, LB-Col; JJC to Asst. Surgeon H. B. Horlbeck, 17 Jun. 1862, LB-Col.

28. JJC to SPM, 8 Apr. 1862, LB-Char.

29. JJC to SPM, 12 Apr. 1862, LB-Char; Supply Table for General and Post Hospitals, *Regulations for the Medical Department of the C.S. Army* (Richmond, Richie & Dunnavant, Printers: 1863) p. 16.

30. Fielding H. Garrison, *An Introduction to the History of Medicine* (Philadelphia, W. B. Saunders Co., 1929), 656; Chisolm, J.J. *A Manual of Military Surgery for*

the Use of Surgeons in the Confederate States Army,1861, 188; JJC to EWJ, 29 May 1862.

31. JJC to Charles Edmondston, 27 May 1962, LB-Col; JJC to EWJ, 29 May 1862, LB-Col.

32. Hasegawa, Guy R. and F. Terry Hambrecht, "The Confederate Medical Laboratories," *Southern Medical Journal*, 96 (December 2003): 1221-1230; JJC to Messrs. J. Asburst & Co, 3 May, 1862, LB-Char; JJC to H. F. Hodson, Esq, 6 Jun. 1862, LB-Col.

33. JJC to EWJ, 4 Aug. 1862, LB-Col; JJC to EWJ, 2 Oct. 1862, LB-Col; George B. Wood and Franklin Bache, *The Dispensatory of the United States of America*, (Philadelphia: J B. Lippincott and Co., 1858).

34. JJC to RAK, 14 Jun. 1862, LB-Col; JJC to EWJ, 19 Jun. 1862, LB-Col; JJC to RAK, 14 Jun. 1862, LB-Col; JJC to Henry B. Horlbeck, 26 Jun. 1862, LB-Col.

35. Hambrecht, F. Terry "Julian John Chisolm," 824.

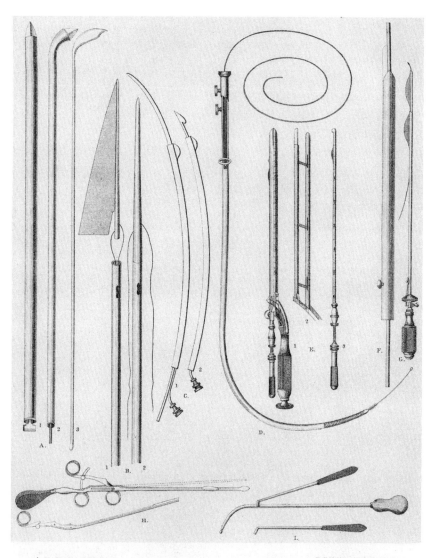

Instruments for procedures involving the urethra
Source: Medical and Surgical History of the War of the Rebellion

- 5 -

"The Privates Were Shot"
Urological Wounds and Treatment
in the Civil War

....

HARRY HERR, M.D.

A soldier was "wounded by a ball in the left of the scrotum, passing backward and wounding the testis, urethra, and rectum." The man was taken from the field on the second day after the fight, and a catheter could not be passed. The urethra near the bulb was laid open, and urine escaped through the scrotum with a greater portion of it exiting by the anus. A gum-elastic catheter was finally passed into the bladder but dispensed with after the fistula closed. The right testis was gone, and the patient suffered persistent urethral fistula, incontinence of urine, severe pain on exercise, and "occasional discharges of matter from the urethra and rectum . . . disability total."

The above report, by Surgeon A. H. Agard and a pension examiner, on a twenty-one-year old private from the 8th Ohio Infantry wounded during the Battle of Cold Harbor, June 3, 1864, gives graphic and grim witness to the debilitating nature of urethral wounds suffered by soldiers during the American Civil War. Although urological injuries were less frequent than the shattered limbs commonly associated with Civil War wounds, they were no less significant. Veterans learned to function and even thrive after the loss of an arm or a leg, but imagine a young man — such as the Ohioan above — facing life soiled in urine and in constant pain, lame from destroyed pelvic bones and nerves, and sexually impotent or mentally scarred by disfigured genitals. Many men survived their pelvic wounds, but sometimes at a terrible cost, leaving many to suffer dire and permanent consequences of their injuries.[1]

Amidst the chaos and pressures of the escalating American Civil War, military surgeons began to observe and record the outcomes of their interventions. In doing so, they established rudimentary standards of care that ultimately saved the lives of a higher proportion of wounded soldiers than their European contemporaries during the Crimean War. This was particularly evident in cases involving injuries of the genitourinary organs. Penetrating wounds of the abdomen, chest, and head were almost always fatal as surgeons did not have the technical expertise to open an abdomen and repair bullet-riddled intestines, stop the bleeding from a gunshot to the lung, or operate safely on an injury to the brain. For those patients, recovery was based more on good fortune than medical know-how.[2]

Pelvic wounds were also considered to be mortal and—in earlier wars—many men suffering such injuries were left to die without receiving any surgical care. Despite this grim conventional wisdom, military surgeons learned how to treat destructive injuries of the kidneys, bladder, urethra, and genitalia during the Civil War, and each year of the war saw improved survival and better recovery.

Understanding the gravity of urological injuries best begins with a study of individual case histories and casualty statistics detailed in the *Medical and Surgical History of the War of the Rebellion* (*MSH*). The study can be supplemented by case studies published by surgeons in the wartime medical literature, military surgeon manuals and handbooks, and—finally—soldier pension files held in the National Archives. Furthermore, army surgeons also performed regular autopsies to better understand the pathology of injuries and why their treatments failed, made drawings of their findings, and submitted specimens to the Army Medical Museum in Washington, D.C.[3]

The Anatomy of a Soldier

A description and illustration of the organs and structures that make up the male genitourinary tract will help the reader understand the detailed descriptions in the following wartime case reports. Briefly, the kidneys and ureters lie in the space behind the abdominal cavity and its contents. The ureters are delicate tubes that conduct urine down from the kidneys to the bladder, located in the pelvis. Urine from the bladder empties into the urethra, which traverses downward through the prostate gland, exits the pelvis and runs through the penis where its channel delivers urine outside the body. The penis is securely attached to the pubic bones by ligaments. The testes are suspended in the scrotum by the spermatic cords, which contain their blood vessels.

Except for the exposed genitals, the urinary organs are relatively well protected in the body from injury. The kidneys are tucked high up underneath the rib cage in front of the large back muscles, and thick bones making up the pelvic girdle surround the bladder and proximal urethra. The location of these organs, however, is both a blessing and a bane. Although serious injury is rendered less common because of their anatomic location, when urinary organs are traumatized, the consequences can be devastating. Urological organs and structures are highly vascular, meaning they bleed profusely when injured, thus risking hemorrhagic shock. Furthermore, when any portion of the urinary tract becomes disrupted, caustic urine escapes into the surrounding tissues, causing substantial damage to soft tissue and bone. Furthermore, the pelvis houses many hidden pockets that provide fertile ground for festering and often fatal abscesses. Urine burrows out through bullet holes, creating urinary fistulas. Even minor wounds can become major problems if they are not recognized and promptly treated.

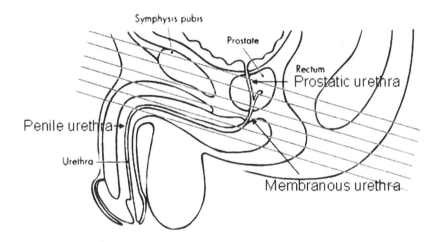

Anatomy of the male urethra. Lines indicate how bullets traversing the pelvis may injure the urethra.

Source: Prepared by Harry Herr, M.D.

It is no wonder, then, that attitudes about pelvic injuries just before the Civil War were grim. Of urological wounds, period medical texts and journals declared matter-of-factly, "injuries of the pelvis must be considered as dangerous as injuries of the head," "death is the most frequent result of shot fractures of the pelvis," and—in the Mexican War—"wounds of the pelvis and parts adjacent were esteemed to be usually fatal."[4]

Likewise, the *Manual of Military Surgery* used by Confederate surgeons regarded the prognosis of pelvic wounds very gloomily, stating, "When portions of the *pelvic parietes* are fractured by heavy projectiles, very protracted abscesses generally arise, connected with necrosed bone. The great force by which these wounds must be produced, and general contusion of the surrounding structures, cause a large proportion, sooner or later, to prove fatal, notwithstanding the peritoneal cavity may have escaped. Even apparently slight cases, as where a portion of the crest of the ileum is carried away by a shell, or ball lodged in the pelvic bones, often prove very tedious from the long-continued exfoliations and abscesses which result."[5]

Confronting the challenges posed by diverse injuries of the urinary and genital organs, the surgeon's knowledge of anatomy, individual judgment, and surgical skill often decided whether a soldier recovered completely, lived with a chronic disability, or suffered a traumatic death.

Injuries of the Kidney and Pelvic Bones

Wartime records categorized the thousands of urological wounds by anatomy: injuries to the kidney, pelvic bones, bladder, rectum, urethra, penis, testis, and other unspecified wounds.

Penetrating gunshot wounds resulted in nearly eighty recorded cases of injury to the kidneys. Shot wounds to the kidney were often associated with fatal wounds of the stomach, liver, spleen, diaphragm, intestines, or spine. Indeed, nearly two-thirds of these men died of hemorrhagic shock or peritonitis from massive kidney wounds. All cases of bilateral renal injury were fatal, while the remainder (about twenty-five cases) recovered from flank wounds to the cortex of the right or left kidney sparing the abdomen.[6]

The least complicated cases occurred when a ball entered the lumbar region and nicked the cortical substance (that is, the outermost or superficial layer of an internal organ). The kidney was implicated by the depth and direction of the wound, bleeding, swelling and pain in the flank, and referred pain in the ipsilateral testicle. If the collecting system was torn, urine mixed with blood escaped by the flank wound. When the peritoneum was lacerated, urine diffused into the abdomen, inevitably causing fatal peritonitis. As opposed to abdominal wounds to the kidney, flank wounds were more likely to recover since bleeding and urine collections, known as urinomas, were isolated, allowing tamponade. Operations to repair or remove injured kidneys were unknown during the war, and army surgeons learned not to disturb flank hemorrhage. A few cases in which a flank wound was probed caused disruption of contained blood clots, usually resulting in fatal hemorrhage.

A case of recovery from a kidney injury is illustrated by a soldier wounded in the last week of the war:

> Private Michael Savilio, Russian, 5th New Hampshire, aged 27 years, was wounded at Farmsville, April 6, 1865, by a round ball, which entered the right 9th rib anteriorly, passed backward and emerged left of the 12th vertebra. Acting Assistant Surgeon Dusenbury reported that for days the patient was confined to bed, complaining of pain in his right testicle. There was slow but steady hemorrhage out the flank wound and into the renal pelvis, which was eliminated in the urine, partly discolored and partly coagulated. The bleeding subsided and pus was seen in the urine, which soon cleared. The wounds healed rapidly and by July 1, he was returned to duty. He was not a pensioner.[7]

This is an excellent example of a flank wound in which blood and urine from the injured kidney eventually stopped under the watchful eye of a diligent surgeon who knew better than to interfere with his patient's capacity to heal his wounds.

There were more than 3,000 cases of gunshot or shell fragment wounds to the pelvis, which fractured one or more pelvic bones or caused significant injury to contained organs, but—interestingly—resulted in only a few minor contusions of the bladder. The bladder was less exposed above the pelvic brim, and surgeons observed that men went into battle with a collapsed bladder owing to dehydration or frequent anxious urinary voiding before their deployment. Tough pelvic bones surrounding an empty bladder protected it from bullet wounds.[8]

Most shot wounds injuring the genitourinary organs or structures involved oblique perforations in which a missile entered the groin, passed through the pelvis and out the buttocks on the opposite side, or struck the hip and traveled across the pelvis in the reverse direction before exiting the opposite groin. Blast shattering of pelvic bone and ricochet of bullets could cause minor or severe injury to urinary organs and adjacent bowel.

Injuries of the Bladder

Nearly 200 cases of direct perforating bullet wounds to the bladder were documented; half of the soldiers died of sepsis owing to extravasation of urine into the peritoneal cavity or surrounding soft tissues, while the remaining half recovered. Surgeons recognized that survival depended on the prompt drainage of urine or the presence of an external urinary fistula to protect the body from infection. In cases of suspected bladder injury, urethral catheters were routinely used. Medical officers' surgical instrument field kits included silver and gum-elastic catheters.[9]

Suprapubic cystotomy (a surgically-created connection between the urinary bladder and the skin) was shunned early in the war because surgeons feared that it facilitated rather than obviated urinary infiltration of surrounding soft tissues, which caused pyogenic suppuration, sepsis, and death. The injured bladder also contracted deep into the pelvis, or was pushed up into the abdomen by hematoma, especially if the bladder neck was disrupted, making it difficult for the surgeon to incise into it above the pubis without risking fatal injury to the bowels. Toward the end of the war, cystotomy was practiced more frequently as surgeons gained experience and operative skills treating bladder injuries and its advantages became more apparent.

Pelvic wounds were probed manually to remove spicules of bone, fragments of bullets, and pieces of clothing, hair, or other foreign objects in the region of the bladder. Bladder fistulas sometimes closed spontaneously after a few weeks with such treatment and the aid of a catheter, but many fistulas persisted for months or years before they healed, often after a piece of bone or even the bullet itself extruded from the external wound or the urethra. Still, complete recoveries of a bladder injury were few, and it was rare to find the functions of the bladder restored to normal after a gunshot wound.[10]

The presence of dead bone was the irritating cause of most persistent urinary fistulas, illustrated by the following case:

> Private C.W., 24th New York, aged 20 years, was wounded at Centreville on August 30, 1862. Acting Assistant Surgeon W. H. Butler reported "a musket ball entered above the pubis ... to the right ... passed obliquely to the left and downward, and escaped . . . above the coccyx." The posterior wound closed, but urine dribbled freely from the anterior one, despite retention of a catheter in the bladder. The catheter proved difficult to pass, "overcome by withdrawing the stylet gradually after the catheter passed under the pubis, and giving it an upward tilt on the inner end." Initially the patient improved, but he developed marked jaundice, became restless and delirious, and died on September 13, 1862. An autopsy showed the ball passed through the left side of the bladder and pieces of bone from the pubis were driven into the bladder. "The walls of the bladder were thickened at least one inch, and its capacity lessened about one-half." Old blood and urine infiltrated the soft tissues of the pelvis around the bladder and there was ulceration of the overlying peritoneum.[11]

Injuries of the Urethra

Of all battle wounds, urethral injuries posed the greatest challenge to army surgeons. Less fatal than kidney or bladder wounds, urethral injury—probably more than other battle wounds, including those necessitating amputation of a limb—was the most troublesome and indeed was most likely to disable injured survivors for the rest of their lives. Dire consequences of a urethral injury included traumatic strictures, urinary fistulas and incontinence, draining abscesses, infection, impotence, chronic pelvic pain, and inability to void without the aid of a catheter. Many men died months and even years later from recurring infections caused by urethral wounds.

Army surgeons suspected urethral injury in cases presenting with blood at the urethral meatus, urinary retention, distended bladder, or intermittent urination through wounds in the perineum, groin, scrotum, penis, or rectum (continuous dribbling of urine from open wounds was felt to be indicative of a bladder injury). In cases of urethral injury, the urogenital diaphragm was recognized as an important anatomic structure. When the urethra was torn below the diaphragm, the scrotum and penis became tremendously swollen and discolored by urine, blood and inflammatory edema. This was a favorable sign for survival, however, because the intact diaphragm contained the urine within the scrotum and prevented it from diffusing up into the pelvis where it could cause fatal abscesses. Absence of scrotal swelling was an ominous sign indicating that the urethra was torn above the diaphragm, discharging urine throughout the pelvis. Surgeons' manuals and handbooks stressed that urethral injuries be treated initially by judicial use of catheters to drain urine to prevent or limit urinary extravasation and by an attempt to realign the lacerated or disrupted urethra with the bladder.[12]

Urethral injures were rarely uncomplicated. Indeed, few of the cases recovered well enough to void without serious difficulty, pain, incontinence, or aid of a catheter. According to pension records, one of every four survivors of urethral injuries required insertion of a catheter to evacuate urine, lived with an indwelling catheter, or wore other cumbersome collecting devices. Others suffered with one or more persistent urethral fistulas associated with total or partial urinary incontinence:

> Private L. J. was wounded at Neuse River February 22, 1865. Surgeon L. W. Reed reported "a gunshot wound of the right natis . . . the ball entered the perineum on the right side, wounding the membranous portion of the urethra, and produced an extensive and almost impassable stricture. A perineal fistula, communicating with the canal, exists, and he passes urine through both fistula and urethra; retention of urine frequently occurs." On May 1, 1872, the examiners of another similarly wounded veteran noted, "He has deep-seated urethro-perineal fistula, and loss of erectile power of the penis, with partial destruction of the left testis, and deformity of the scrotum. . . . The disability is no doubt permanent. There is constant dribbling of urine, which produces excoriation of the parts, and in warm weather gives rise to an exceedingly offensive odor; disability total."[13]

Injuries of the Penis and Testis

These were not rare; more than 300 shot wounds to the penis were reported and at least one bayonet wound, ranging from mostly minor wounds of the prepuce or shaft to partial or total amputation. Very few of these cases were uncomplicated. The most frequently associated injuries were wounds to the scrotum and testes, perineum and thighs, and pelvic walls or viscera. Forty-one cases terminated fatally, usually from associated injuries to the pelvis or intercurrent infection. Debridement of the wound was the rule, and surgical amputation of a traumatized penis was rare. On several occasions, projectiles were extracted from the corpora, but only "in a virile organ of extraordinary dimensions." Erections hindered healing, and sexual excitement was to be "sedulously avoided." Camphor enemas were used and the patient was exhorted to "shun lascivious thoughts."[14]

Only two self-inflicted knife wounds of the penis in insane soldiers were noted, but there were several instances of similar injuries occurring in brothels, one luckless subject having his penis maliciously amputated.[15]

Perhaps less frequent than anticipated from their exposed position, a total of nearly 600 cases of testicular injury from missiles was recorded, mostly contusions or lacerations The gonads are partially protected from serious injury by a tough capsular tunic. Wounds of the testis commonly caused acute pain, radiating to the loins, and were generally attended by faintness and vomiting. Most recovered, but a small percentage died, complicated by wounds to the pelvis, thigh, and perineum.[16]

Cases were treated by orchiectomy (removal of the testis, or castration). Surprisingly, no bayonet wounds to the testis were reported. Testis injury often resulted in subsequent atrophy, testicular pain (orchalgia), hydrocele formation, and impotence.

> Private J. B., 9th Maine, aged eighteen years, was wounded at Fort Wagner, July 18, 1863. Surgeon D. Merritt reported, "gunshot wound of the external genitals; a minie ball, tearing open the scrotum on the right side . . . passed through the thigh . . . and was extracted, on the field, from the gluteal muscles. Had the testicle been put in the scrotum and sutures used, thereby closing the scrotum, the result of the case might have been different; but after waiting a few days, and applying cool and soothing lotions, the resulting condition was such that invited surgeons and myself deemed an operation was necessary, and castration was accordingly performed."[17]

The surgeon was probably right that debridement of the devitalized portion of the scrotum and primary closure might have preserved the testis. Later, however, when it became clear that gangrene was imminent, orchiectomy saved the boy's life.

Traumatic injury of the genitals presaged depression, and many pensioners were noted to have melancholy thoughts and suicidal tendencies. More than a hundred cases with "loss of virile power" or "impotence" were mentioned in association with injuries of the testis or penis. The frequency of erectile dysfunction was probably much greater, especially after the war from posttraumatic stress. Recognition of war-caused mental health problems began during the Civil War, but serious research into physical and mental health costs of traumatic war experiences among Civil War veterans is just now beginning.[18]

Catheters: Use, Disuse, and Misuse

Catheters have been used since antiquity to relieve urinary passages blocked by disease, but they emerged as essential life-saving devices during the Civil War. Catheterization of the bladder was regarded as indispensable in wounds of the bladder and urethra and became the established rule of practice during the war. For example, Confederate surgeon J. J. Chisolm wrote, "the catheter should be introduced as soon as possible after the reception of the wound and should be worn continuously for four or five days, until adhesive inflammation has closed the torn cellular tissue, and shut up the avenues into which the urine would have escaped. If a catheter cannot be passed into the bladder a free incision should be made through the perineum for evacuation of urine."[19]

Likewise, the *Medical and Surgical History* related important lessons learned during the war, stating, "The immediate introduction of a catheter after a shot laceration of the urethra will often present great difficulties to the field surgeon, pressed for time and unprovided with a variety of catheters. Nevertheless, the attempt must be made, with the utmost caution and delicacy of manipulation, without waiting until the desire to urinate is urgent."[20]

The catheters used during the Civil War were made of silver metal, gutta-percha (a tough, rubberlike gum), or gum-elastic (silken-thread frame coated with a mixture of linseed oil and a hard, lustrous gum resin called copal). They were curved (made to follow the curve of the male urethra up into the bladder) and came in various sizes and shapes, with one or two side holes recessed from a conical, olivary or cylindrical tip.

Caoutchouc vulcanized rubber catheters were also used, especially toward the end of the war. Catheters made of this substance were softer and more pliable than rigid metal or gum-elastic catheters (which were actually stiff in spite of their name), and they were much better tolerated in cases of self-catheterization or if continuous catheter drainage was required for more than a few days.[21]

To be sure, there were problems and errors during the war. Unsterilized catheters were reused, there was no lubricating jelly available to ease their passage, and — despite the prevailing wisdom — some surgeons continued to counsel against their use. Still, the record is undeniable; when a catheter was successfully inserted into the bladder, cases with a satisfactory outcome outnumbered unsatisfactory results by more than five to one. Indeed the use of a catheter could be the differences between life and death: infiltration of urine into the surrounding soft tissues could cause fatal sepsis.

Successful catheterization under difficult circumstances required time, patience, skill, and more than a little luck. The procedure was considered so important by army surgeons they frequently administered chloroform to calm a flailing patient. How long to leave a catheter in the injured urethra was determined by attendant circumstances: from as little as twenty four hours to prolonged use until the wound showed signs of healing. Surgeons believed the gravity of infection from undrained urine far outweighed the harm caused by prolonged retention of a catheter. If a catheter could not be inserted into the bladder, the surgeon attempted to introduce a filiform (made of gum or whalebone). Often even the smallest catheter could not be passed, and surgeons were advised to avoid the hazard of creating false passages by forced catheterization.

The following wartime case study illustrates application of sound surgical principles resulting in a reasonably favorable outcome with judicious use of catheters:

> Private J. R., 8th Infantry, age 27, was wounded, February 2, 1865. Several surgeons reported shot wound of left buttock, exiting "through the scrotum, destroying the right testis. The perineum and right groin were much ecchymosed and swollen. Urine passed in small quantity through the perineal opening. The urethra was severed in the membranous portion. . . . At mid-day no urine passed and the bladder was much

distended." After unsuccessful attempts at catheterization, the bladder was punctured above the pubes, thirty-five ounces of urine were drawn off, and "a catheter was kept in the bladder through this opening for two days, when, through the carelessness of the attendants, it was allowed to come out. Then the urine escaped through the wound in the urethra." A perineal section and urethrotomy was practiced, through which a silver catheter was placed for the purpose of restoring the urine to its natural course through the urethra. No urine escaped through the perineal opening for 14 days while the catheter remained in the urethra. When it was removed, urine "again took its old passage through the wound in the urethra" until February 8, 1866, when the fistula closed after the urethra was kept open by daily passage of a gum-elastic catheter. The urine "never returned to its unnatural outlet through the fistula in the urethra. . . . He is now able to retain the urine at will; when he voids . . . the urine mostly passes by the urethra, but a portion sometimes escapes through the perineal opening."[22]

Chronic urethral fistulas were particularly problematic, and definitive surgical treatment was nonexistent. Cauterization and primary suture to close urethral fistulas were attempted, but such measures virtually always failed. The following case illustrates the best efforts of surgeons unknowingly thwarted by an unwitting paramour.

Case A. P.F., aged twenty-one years was left with "two fistules of the membranous urethra, the result of a severe lacerated wound of the perineum. Assistant Surgeon W. Thomson "pared the edges of the apertures and approximated them by silver sutures. A catheter was retained in the bladder, the urethra having been dilated freely by the daily use of bougies. . . . The posterior orifice appeared to have closed; but it reopened, and recourse was again had to cauterization, without advantage. There was such loss of substance, nearly a third of the cylinder of the urethra being destroyed, that the restoration of the canal was a very difficult problem. After a few weeks, the callous edges of the fistules were again refreshed and approximated by sutures, which soon tore out, and it was discovered that the patient had received visits after this, as after the former operation, from a young woman to whom he was affianced, whose tender ministrations induced a local hyperemia very prejudicial to the success of any plastic procedure."[23]

Various, and often ingenious, methods of urethroplasty, using penile and scrotal flaps, were tried. These were seldom successful, but they provided the impetus for staged repairs to come. Modern urethroplasty techniques would not evolve for another fifty years.

Lessons Learned

Surgeons treated nearly 1,500 cases of urological injury during the American Civil War. They did so without knowledge of germ theory or antisepsis, and without intravenous fluids, blood products, antibiotics, sterile equipment, monitoring gauges, or x-rays. They operated outside—often in field hospitals—using crude instruments under inadequate lighting and without trained anesthesiologists or nurses. Water was in short supply to quench the thirst of the wounded, to wash the surgeons' hands, or to clean their instruments. Given these conditions, infection became the surgeons' and soldiers' worst enemy.

Still—even working against these odds—army surgeons learned quickly and worked hard to improve their techniques. Every year the war was fought, they gained a greater understanding of the magnitude of war wounds and their potential consequences, refined their interventions appropriately, and saw their results improve. For example, when considering all gunshot wounds to the pelvis each year of the war, nearly twice as many men survived and recovered from urological injuries during the last two years compared to those who sustained similar injuries during the first and second year.[24]

The lack of appropriate instruments, as we know them today, was a major problem. Metal catheters were stiff and dangerous in that they could make false pathways instead of finding the correct one. The gum elastic catheter was superior, but it also was stiff and inflexible. Even when the bladder and urethra were successfully instrumented for urine drainage, the catheter could not be left in place for long due to recognized calculus and stricture formation, which began within a few days or weeks. Surgeons faced the conundrum that protracted retention of a catheter in the urethra for more than four or five days could retard healing and cause a troublesome stricture or fistula as well as difficulty in replacing it when removed. In severe injuries, a filiform was often left in the bladder as a guide to permit introduction of open-ended soft rubber catheters repeatedly as necessary. Many of the injured were taught intermittent self-catheterization.

Although perineal urethrotomy was used successfully for wounds to the bulbar urethra or partial disruptions of the bladder neck, the urethra was left open to allow secondary healing. While this procedure undoubtedly saved lives and worked early on, as the wound began to heal, scar formation usually caused a severe stricture at the injured site obstructing the free flow of urine. If dilation of the surgically created opening was not performed regularly, chronic retention and overflow incontinence of urine led to ascending urinary infection and eventual uremia, suggesting that kidney failure probably caused many deaths years after the injury.

Today's initial management of bladder and urethral injuries focuses on primary repair and suprapubic cystostomy for urinary diversion. Although the *Medical and Surgical History* records a few cases in which suprapubic puncture was used, it was not until World War I that the importance of suprapubic diversion was realized as a preferred and essential life-saving measure for pelvic and lower urinary tract injuries. Review of individual cases from the Civil War illustrates that the procedure probably could have saved many soldiers who ultimately died from infection and would have minimized subsequent traumatic effects owing to frequent perineal and urethral catheterizations. Army surgeons were justifiably cautious, however, because finding the injured bladder was difficult, catheters were not available for long-term intubation, and incising into the belly by mistake usually proved fatal.

A number of urological advances emerged from the Civil War. Surgeons learned to avoid disturbing a contained flank hematoma in a stable patient (even today, expectant management is still the preferred method of handling kidney trauma). They learned the gravity of shot wounds to the pelvis had been exaggerated in the European medical literature. Treated vigorously and attended to daily, pelvic injuries actually caused far less mortality than abdominal wounds. Whereas more than three-quarters of abdominal wounds were fatal, an equal proportion of pelvic injuries recovered, even those involving the rectum. Surgeons learned when and how to debride devitalized tissue, control hemorrhage, and provide drainage of urine in the pelvis by using urethral catheters, perineal urethrotomy when necessary, and on rare occasions, suprapubic cystostomy. Exteriorizing urine (and feces) improved the chances of recovery. Surgeons learned the importance and advantage of removing dead bone and other foreign bodies from the bladder or urethra to promote and hasten healing. They also questioned the propriety of leaving a catheter for too long in the urethra, observing that this often worsened, and even caused, urethral injury, leaving many cases with permanent urethral fistula and stricture. Intermittent catheterization became common practice. They realized that castration was sometimes hastily resorted to unwisely, and they tried to repair injured testes (and penis) knowing that genital injuries carried traumatic and devastating consequences beyond the wound itself. They noted the time from injury to receiving definitive surgical care (a catheter) averaged an astonishing five days, undoubtedly causing some premature deaths and complicating recovery in others.

The war provided a fertile training ground for a large number of under-educated and inexperienced physicians. As surgeons acquired experience during the war, they exercised better judgment and devised and tested new surgical methods to save and rehabilitate more men. Most important, after the war they began to organize medical societies to learn from each other's experiences and debate the best methods of treatments. Civil War surgeons extracted the most information that they could from meticulous observations, published medical papers and educated others. An outstanding example was Confederate surgeon Hunter H. McGuire, who published his experiences, educated others by founding a medical school, and became president of the American Medical Association. Civil War surgeons also helped found the American College of Surgeons, and the first and still most prestigious scientific urological society extant today, the American Association of Genitourinary Surgeons. The end result was a remarkably improved quality of American medicine as a whole.

Richard Turner-Warwick, the renowned British surgeon, probably put it best, stating, "It is the urologist who has to share the burden of the ultimate urologic disability with the patient when the thoracic, the abdominal, and even the orthopedic aspects are long forgotten." His words ring true, then and now.[25]

Notes

1. *The Medical and Surgical History of the Civil War* (Reprint, 13 Volumes, 2 Volume Index, Wilmington, N.C.: Broadfoot Publishing Co., 1992), Vol. 9: 370. The pagination for this volume corresponds to that used in vol. 2, pt. 2, ch. 7 ("Injuries to the Pelvis") of the original *Medical and Surgical History of the War of the Rebellion*.

2. *Medical and Surgical History of the British Army Which Served in Turkey and the Crimea During the War Against Russia in the Years 1854-55-56* (London, 1858), 335.

3. *The Medical and Surgical History of the War of the Rebellion* (2 Volumes, 6 Parts Each, Washington, DC: Government Printing Office, 1870-88).

4. L. Stromeyer, *Maximen der Kriegsheilkunst* (Hanover, 1855): 655; Carl Ferdinand Lohmeyer, *Die Schusswunden und ihre Behandlung Kurz bearb* (Gottingen: Wigand, 1859):147; J. B. Porter, "Surgical Notes of the Mexican War," *American Journal of the Medical Sciences*, 23 (1852), 30.

5. J. J. Chisolm, *A Manual of Military Surgery Prepared for the Use of Surgeons in the Confederate States Army* (Richmond: West & Johnson, 1861):61.

6. J. A. Lidell, "Injuries of Abdominal Viscera by Firearms," *American Journal of the Medical Sciences*, 53 (1867), 356; C. H. Carpenter, "Fatal Kidney Injuries," *Boston Medical and Surgical Journal*, 71 (1865), 112.

7. H. Dusenbury, "Cases of Gunshot Wounds of the Abdomen Involving Viscera," *American Journal of the Medical Sciences*, 50 (1865), 400.

8. *Medical and Surgical History of the Civil War*, Vol. 12: 168.

9. Charles S. Tripler and George C. Blackman, *Handbook for the Military Surgeon* (Cincinnati: Robert Clarke & Co., 1861): ii.

10. *Medical and Surgical History of the Civil War*, Vol. 9: 255.

11. Ibid, p. 291.

12. J. J. Chisolm, *A Manual of Military Surgery Prepared for the Use of Surgeons in the Confederate States Army* (Columbia, SC: Evans & Cogswell, 1864): 352.

13. *Medical and Surgical History of the Civil War*, Vol. 9: 364.

14. Frank H. Hamilton, "Gunshot Wounds of the Penis," *American Medical Times*, 9 (1864), 61; *Medical and Surgical History of the Civil War*, Vol. 9: 346-47.

15. *Medical and Surgical History of the Civil War*, Vol. 9: 344.

16. J. Homans, "Gunshot Wounds of the Testes," *Boston Medical and Surgical Journal*, 72 (1865), 15; Frank H. Hamilton, "Gunshot Wounds of the Scrotum and Testes," *American Medical Times*, 9 (1864), 61.

17. *Medical and Surgical History of the Civil War*, Vol. 9: 415.

18. Judith Pizarro, Roxane Cohen Silver, and JoAnn Prause, "Physical and Mental Health Costs of Traumatic War Experiences Among Civil War Veterans," *Archives of General Psychiatry*, 63 (February 2006), 193-200.

19. J. J. Chisolm, *A Manual of Military Surgery* (1864): 352.

20. *Medical and Surgical History of the Civil War,* Vol. 9: 381.

21. H. J. Bigelow, "Urethral Catheters," *Boston Medical and Surgical Journal*, 40 (1849), 9.

22. *Medical and Surgical History of the Civil War,* Vol. 9: 365.

23. Ibid, 402.

24. Ibid, 342.

25. Richard Turner-Warwick, personal communication.

Confederate States of America.

MEDICAL PURVEYOR'S OFFICE,

Savannah, September 8th. 1862.

The following named Indigenous Remedies are wanted by the Medical Department, for which the annexed prices will be paid. To be delivered at either of my Offices in Savannah or Macon, properly dried and in good order, labeled, and each, when practicable, containing a dried specimen of the whole plant.

	Per Pound.		Per Pound.
Arum Triphyllum, Root, (Indian Turnip, or Wake Robin)	$ 30	Iris Versicolor, root, (Blue Flag,)	30
Asclepias Tuberosa, Root, (Pleurisy or Butterfly Weed Root)	25	Juglans Cinerea, leaves and inner bark of root, (Butternut,)	50
Aristolcchia Serpentaria, Root, (Virginia Snake Root)	1 00	Lobelia Inflata, seeds, (Lobelia)	1 50
Arctostaphylos Uva Ursi, Leaves, (Uva Ursi)	30	" " herb, "	50
Arctium Lappa, Root, (Burdock)	20	Leptandra Virginica, root, (Black Root, Culver's Physic)	50
" " Seeds, "	20	Laurus Sassafras, red, bark of root, (Sassafras)	30
Asarum Canadense, Root, (Wild Ginger or Colts Foot, &c.)	50	Liquidambar Styraciflua, inner bark, (Sweet Gum Tree)	10.
Apocynum Androsemifolium, Root, (Bitter Root)	40	" " resin, " "	1 00
" Cannabinum, Root, (Indian Hemp)	50	Myrica Cerifera, bark of root, (Low Bush Myrtle)	35
Acorus Calamus, root, (Calamus)	25	Mentha Piperita, herb, (Peppermint)	30
Cimicifuga Racemosa, root, (Black Cohosh)	50	" Viridis, " (Spearmint)	25
Corallorhiza Odontorhiza, root, (Crawley)	2 00	Nymphæa Odorata, root, (White Pond Lilly)	10
Cypripedium Pubescens, root, (Lady's Slipper)	1 00	Polygala Senega, root, (Seneca Snake Root)	1 00
Convallaria Multiflora, root, (Solomon's Seal)	30	Prunus Virginiana, bark, (Wild Cherry Tree)	30
Corydalis Formosa, root, (Turkey Corn, Wild Turkey Pea)	50	Podophyllum Peltatum, root, (Mandrake)	30
Chionanthus Virginica, bark of root, (Fringe Tree)	30	Panax Quinquefolium, root, (Ginseng)	50
Chimaphila Umbellata, whole plant, (Pipssewa)	30	Pinckneya Pubens, inner bark,	30
Chelone Glabra, leaves and small twigs, (Balmony)	50	Phytolacca Decandra, berries, (Poke)	30
Conium Maculatum, leaves and seeds, (Poison Hemlock)	25	Rhus Glabra, berries, (Sumach Berries)	15
Chenopodium Anthelminticum, seeds. (Jerusalem Oak)	25	Ricinus Communis, seeds, (Palma Christi) per bushel	7 00
Capsicum of all kinds, (Red Pepper)	1 00	Sanguinaria Canadensis, root, (Blood Root) per pound	50
Euphorbia Ipecacuanha, bark of root, (Wild Ipecac)	50	Symphytum Officinale, root, (Comfrey)	25
Eupatorium Perfoliatum, small twigs. leaves and flowers,		Sinapis Alba, seeds, (White Mustard)	75
(Boneset)	30	" Nigra, " (Black Mustard)	75
Eupatorium Purpurium, root, (Queen of the Meadow,)	50	Stillingia Sylvatica, root, (Queens Delight)	20
Geranium Maculatum, root, (Cranesbill or Crowfoot)	1 00	Salix, inner bark, (Willow)	30
Gelseminum Sempervirens, root, (Yellow Jessamine)	25	Spigelia Marilandica, root, (Pink Root)	30
Hyoscyamus Nigra, leaves and seeds, (Henbane)	50	Ulmus Fulva, inner bark (Slippery Elm)	30
Hydrastis Canadensis, root, (Golden Seal,)	1 00	Veratrum Viride, root, (American Hellebore)	25
Hamamelis Virginica, leaves, (Witch Hazel)	30	Xanthoxylum Fraxineum, bark, (Prickly Ash)	30
" " bark of shrub, "	30	" " berries, "	50

W. H. PRIOLEAU,

Ass't Surg. P. A. C. S., and Medical Purveyor 4th Depot.

Handbill asking Southern citizens to collect medicinal plants for the army.

Source: Record Group 109, Entry 30, National Archives and Records Administration, Washington, D.C.

Southern Resources, Southern Medicines

GUY R. HASEGAWA, PHARM.D.

Historians recognize that one of the Confederate Army's most note-worthy accomplishments in dealing with the Union blockade was providing its troops with sufficient arms and ammunition to carry on a long and hard-fought war. Less well known is the story, summarized here, of how the same army marshaled a wide array of resources, natural and otherwise, to furnish its physicians with the medicines needed to treat the vast numbers of sick and wounded soldiers.[1]

The Confederate medical department's wish list for drugs was its standard supply table for hospitals, which duplicated almost exactly its Union counterpart and included an array of medicines, from acacia to zinc sulfate. Unfortunately, the conditions in the North that allowed for an uninterrupted supply of the items—a continued influx of goods from abroad and the capacity for large-scale drug manufacturing—were not as easy for the South to replicate. Some medicines in the table, like fluid extract of wild cherry bark, were made from plants growing in North America, but many others, like quinine, originated in foreign lands. Moreover, drugs like mercurial compounds, chloroform, and ether, which were made from minerals or chemicals, were not being produced in large amounts in the nonindustrial South. Before the war, these circumstances dictated that the South obtain its drugs from overseas or from Northern dealers or manufacturers. The onset of hostilities and the reduction of trade with the North forced Confederate Army supply officers, called medical purveyors, to rely initially on purchases from blockade runners and local druggists and medical wholesalers. (It is ironic that the war also threatened to cut off the supply of Southern plants needed by Northern physicians.) Although foreign goods arrived in Southern ports fairly frequently early in the war, a tightening blockade, a prolonged conflict, and rising drug prices—driven by scarcity, inflation, and speculators—would spell trouble for an army that needed massive quantities of medicines.[2]

These prospects, soon to become realities, led Army Surgeon General Samuel Preston Moore to conclude before the war was a year old that the South itself should be tapped as a well of supplies for his surgeons. Thus, orders for manufactured items — cots, tourniquets, and surgical instruments, for instance — were placed with local businesses and artisans, and natural resources, especially plants, were turned into medicines. The objects behind the "appropriation of our indigenous medicinal substances of the vegetable kingdom," announced Moore, were to take greater advantage of the South's resources and reduce its payment for foreign goods. (In this context, "indigenous" plants included species native to the Confederate states as well as those introduced into the South from other lands.) In practical terms, Moore hoped that Southern drug production would supplement other sources of supply such that the army would have sufficient medicines for its needs.[3]

The Decision to Use Southern Plants

An important undercurrent to the Confederate medical department's situation was the friction between allopathic ("regular" or orthodox) physicians and other practitioners. Most Confederate surgeons, including Surgeon General Moore, were allopaths. A number of medical sects disapproved of the harsh drugs and other "heroic" treatments, such as bloodletting, used by some allopaths and instead advocated relatively mild remedies, often derived from North American flora. Allopaths already knew about and prescribed some of those plants, but they often regarded botanical and other sectarian practitioners as quacks and rejected their teachings as irrational.[4]

After the war, Moore explained his decision to turn to indigenous flora: "It had been my impression for a long time that many of the Southern medicinal plants possessed valuable properties, and that their usefulness would soon be discovered in many diseases if administered with care and attention." Moore may have dismissed the views of botanical practitioners, but his lack of certainty about the plants' value also seems, at first glance, to indicate a distrust of the established allopathic knowledge base. Among the species eventually used by the Confederate army, the vast majority were already in *The Pharmacopoeia of the United States of America* (*USP*), the standard listing of allopathic drugs. Many were described in the prewar curricula of Southern allopathic medical schools, such as the Atlanta

Medical College and the Medical College of the State of South Carolina. Large numbers of future Confederate surgeons attended Northern medical schools like the University of Pennsylvania, whose materia medica course covered dozens of medicinal plants growing in the South. Some allopathic physicians studied and published articles about native plants.[5]

Credible information, however, did not necessarily give physicians confidence in remedies they did not personally prescribe. Moore had served in the United States Army as a surgeon for twenty-six years and may have had little opportunity to use remedies that were not on the army's standard list. Even practitioners familiar with Southern plants in civilian practice had little idea of the medicines' value in treating the maladies of a large army. Whereas the allopathic literature described the medicinal properties of native plants, it did not generally claim that they surpassed or even matched standard drugs in value. Thus, it is understandable that Moore's views about the usefulness of indigenous plants formed not a conviction but rather an impression, albeit one that clearly required action.[6]

The first known step of the surgeon general's office in promoting the use of native flora was its publication on March, 21, 1862, of a pamphlet of indigenous medicinal plants, which was distributed to medical officers on April 2. There was good reason at the time to fear that the flow of goods from abroad was in jeopardy. Just a few months earlier, in November 1861, a Union victory at Port Royal Sound, South Carolina, had provided the U.S. Navy with a splendid base for blockading operations. During the same month, Union forces had occupied Tybee Island, Georgia, a move that threatened Fort Pulaski, which guarded the sea approach to Savannah. The pamphlet listed sixty-seven of the South's "more important medicinal plants" and described where they grew and their uses, formulations, and dosage. Moore maintained control over the selection of plants and instructed his surgeons to collect the listed species and send them to medical purveyors. He also directed medical officers to investigate the value of indigenous remedies in relieving pain or inducing vomiting or defecation, because of the relatively small number of Southern plants recognized as useful for those purposes.[7]

In a circular issued on July 22, 1862, Moore reminded surgeons of the uses of several indigenous medicinal plants and encouraged them to report on the antimalarial effectiveness of *Pinckneya pubens* (Georgia bark), which had not been mentioned in the recent pamphlet. By the summer of 1862, medical purveyors were already issuing substitutes in place of scarce standard items, and this sometimes displeased the recipients. "The Surgeons around here," wrote a medical purveyor to his assistant, "expect what they order whether it is in the Confederacy or not. They cannot appreciate kindness in substituting one medicine for another rather than let them go without."[8]

F. P. Porcher and the Selection of Plants

How Moore identified the plants most worthy of initial attention is unclear. Since several standard medicines were made from species that grew in the South, collecting those species was an obvious first step. But what about the other plants listed in the pamphlet? Historians usually credit an 1863 book by physician-botanist Francis Peyre Porcher with bringing useful native plants to the attention of medical officers—-the work was hailed after the war as having "saved the Confederacy for two years"—but clearly it could not have influenced the decisions that Moore made by March 1862.[9]

Porcher was a surgeon for the Holcombe Legion of South Carolina volunteers before Moore directed him on March 11, 1862, to command the General Hospital at Fort Nelson, near Norfolk, Virginia. This was a choice posting but had no clear connection with Porcher's botanical expertise. At some point, the surgeon general recognized that Porcher would be an apt appointee to compile information about indigenous flora. Moore may have been convinced of this after reading Porcher's August 1861 article in *De Bow's Review*—Porcher had given him a copy—which urged Southern self-sufficiency and described about thirty Southern plants with medicinal value. Porcher may also have been recommended for the task by Surgeon J. J. Chisolm, medical purveyor at Charleston, South Carolina, who knew Porcher well and wrote frequently to the surgeon general.[10]

On May 27, 1862, shortly after the Confederates evacuated Norfolk, Moore ordered Porcher to establish a botanical garden and "enlarge the [1862] pamphlet," which the surgeon general thought "did not meet the requirements of the army or the necessities of the people of the Confederacy." Moore's written orders did not direct Porcher to identify additional medicinal plants. In fact, the surgeon general told a medical purveyor less than four months later that "respecting the use of the Indigenous Remedies of the South, it is not desirable that the list of articles employed should be multiplied." Thus, Moore may have wanted Porcher to limit himself to supplying more details about the plants already selected. "After your *pamphlet* [emphasis added] shall have been finished," Moore told Porcher on June 10, 1862, "and the garden in operation, you can be assigned to hospital duty." Porcher had made a point in his *De Bow's* article to highlight Georgia bark as worth studying, and this may have accounted for the surgeon general encouraging its investigation as early as July 1862. Moore may also have been influenced to mention Georgia bark by a report from Medical Purveyor William Prioleau, who had heard about the plant's supposed effectiveness and was taking steps to collect it.[11]

The result of Porcher's labors, available as early as March 1863, was not a pamphlet but a 601-page book reviewing the literature on Southern natural resources with potential medicinal and other uses. The book, *Resources of the Southern Fields and Forests*, was in some ways an expanded version of Porcher's *De Bow's* article; the same major title was used in both works, and neither was confined to medical topics. The length and organization of the book—sections were arranged according to the plants' taxonomic classification—probably did little to make it a user-friendly guide to the selection, preparation, and administration of indigenous remedies. Its scholarly nature, though, and the fact that it was compiled by Porcher, a respected allopath, may have convinced some medical officers that reliable evidence supported the plants' use. Without such credentials, a book urging the use of native flora might have been viewed by allopaths as promoting the doctrine of some fringe group of botanical practitioners.[12]

Coinciding with the publication of Porcher's book in the spring of 1863 was the issuance by the surgeon general's office of the standard supply table of indigenous remedies, which listed the remedies' uses and dosages and the amounts to be issued. The table included sixty-five plants, only seven of which had not already appeared in the 1862 pamphlet; the most important addition was probably Georgia bark. In a preface to the table, Moore called Porcher's book a source of "much reliable information," and the surgeon general occasionally referred medical officers to the book in subsequent communications. A circular issued by the surgeon general's office in April 1863 specified that "when the articles of the original Supply Table called for are not on hand, or are deficient in quantity, Medical Purveyors are instructed to exercise their discretion in substituting such of the Indigenous articles and in such quantities as may supply the deficiencies."[13]

At least thirty indigenous plants other than those listed in the table of indigenous remedies were eventually collected and issued by medical purveyors—presumably with Moore's blessing—but only a handful of species accounted for the bulk of such agents used by Confederate surgeons. This was consistent with Moore's position that it was more important to identify a few of the most useful plants in various therapeutic classes than to simply add more species to the list of possible remedies. Indeed, it would have been difficult for allopathically trained surgeons to master the use of scores of indigenous remedies with which they were previously unfamiliar, so limiting the number of plants collected and issued made good sense both logistically and clinically.[14]

Other Influences on Plant Selection

If Porcher's major and possibly sole contribution to the army's selection of indigenous plants was his persuading the surgeon general to endorse Georgia bark, then other possible influences on Moore's choices were the standard medical literature, testimony by trusted medical officers, and advice from medical sects that favored botanical treatment.

A standard drug reference of the day for allopaths was *The Dispensatory of the United States of America* (*USD*), one of only two books that remained throughout the war in the Confederate standard supply table for hospitals. The massive and highly informative *USD*, revised every several years, described the sources, constituents, properties, and uses of the hundreds of articles listed in the *USP*. It also included an appendix of "drugs not recognized by the American or British Pharmacopoeias, yet possessing some interest from their former or existing relations to Medicine and Pharmacy." It did not, however, help in the selection of treatments for specific ailments. Nearly all of the plants known to have been sought by Confederate medical purveyors appeared in the well-referenced book, and it was relied upon by the purveyors for information about the identification and preparation of the plants. All sixty-five plants in the standard supply table of indigenous remedies appeared in the 1858 *USD*: thirty-eight as primary *USP* drugs, twenty-four as secondary *USP* drugs, and three in the appendix. In hindsight, it seems that the *USD* could have assisted Moore in plant selection as well as any other single source available during the war. He evidently considered it inadequate in some respect, or he would not have given Porcher the assignment he did. For physicians, the *USD*'s most important drawback, compared with Porcher's book, was probably its lack of an index of drug uses.[15]

Allopathic medical journals of the time often carried reports of the usefulness of nonstandard medicines, many of which were derived from Southern plants. Porcher, for instance, published in 1849 a detailed report on the medicinal flora of South Carolina, and in September 1861, scientist and future Confederate surgeon Joseph Jones published a lengthy article urging the examination of Southern flora and reviewing plants that might be useful in the treatment of malaria. The extent to which Moore consulted or relied on such resources is uncertain. One remedy that received a fair amount of attention in journals and the *USD* as a treatment for malaria was cottonseed tea, yet there is no evidence that cottonseed, which should have been plentiful in the South, was ever considered for use in the Confederate Army. On the other hand, Moore—on the basis, evidently, of one surgeon's enthusiastic endorsement—directed medical officers to try treating malaria with external applications of turpentine, even though the therapy was mentioned only rarely in the literature.[16]

Moore required a delicate touch in dealing with botanical practitioners. He would have had no trouble getting clinical advice from them, but many Confederate surgeons would probably have resisted any action that they perceived as an adoption of the sectarians' principles and remedies. That the surgeon general anticipated skepticism about the plants' use is evident in his appeal to medical officers to "lay aside all prejudice which may exist in their minds against their use, and ... give them a fair opportunity for the exhibition of their remedial virtues which they certainly possess." Indeed, sentiment toward indigenous remedies, at least among medical purveying personnel, was sometimes disparaging. Medical Purveyor Prioleau's chief chemist contemptuously referred to persons collecting plants for the medical department as "root diggers," and a hospital steward who had worked in the Richmond purveying office thought indigenous plants sat "like a nightmare upon the brain of the Surgeon General."[17]

Moore, realizing the need for practical assistance with native plants, hired botanical physician William T. Park, a member of the "reform" medical sect and a trustee of the Southern Reform Medical College in Macon, Georgia, to help Medical Purveyor Prioleau collect and process Southern plants. Moore and Park disagreed about the plants that should be gathered, and Park, subsequently dismissed from his position, cited Moore's alleged "antipathy to the Reform Profession." Prioleau later worked closely with Methvin S. Thomson, who was also a trustee of the Southern Reform Medical College and a professor of materia medica and other subjects at that institution. Thomson helped Prioleau construct a laboratory for drug production and used his own grinding apparatus to pulverize native plants that Prioleau had gathered. It appears that any assistance that the army medical department accepted from botanical practitioners was limited to the identification, collection, and processing of plants that Moore had already determined should be used.[18]

Collection of Resources

Some medicinal plants could be used with minimal or no processing—a simple preparation of the easily collected common elder, for example, was supposedly useful for expelling maggots from wounds—so soldiers sometimes harvested flora for their own surgeons or hospitals. At other times, soldier-gathered plants were forwarded to medical purveyors for further preparation. Medical purveyors published newspaper advertisements and handbills offering payment to citizens for the collection and delivery of listed plants. Medical Purveyor Chisolm in South Carolina reported that the conscription laws and volunteering for the army would leave few healthy men to collect plants and that the "parties most likely to aid in this matter were the wives and children of soldiers in service." He suggested that the surgeon general establish "a district Bureau for the collection of indigenous plants under the charge of Surg F P Porcher whose tastes and occupation has long made familiar with such duties"; Porcher never received such an assignment. One purveyor even tried to enlist circuit riders to spread the word that plants were needed. Amassing adequate quantities of plants was a challenge, especially if the purveyor was unfamiliar with the plants or with what they were worth. Medical Purveyor Prioleau admitted, "As I am not at all conversant with the appearance of these plants I would like very much to have some one who understands them." Prioleau found the assistance of botanical physicians Park and Thomson useful, and these consultants sometimes acted as agents through whom Prioleau purchased plants.[19]

Most species used by the Confederacy were found growing wild, but Southern women were encouraged to cultivate poppies and deliver the raw opium to medical purveyors. Other growers supplied castor beans. Corn and other grains were used by distillers to manufacture whiskey, which was purchased by the medical department for administration to patients or preparing medicines. The Confederate medical department attempted the large-scale cultivation of poppies, flax, and black mustard.[20]

Plants were not the only resources used by the medical department. Sulfur and iron pyrites were gathered from mines and used in the production of sulfuric acid, which was needed to produce chloroform, ether, and other drugs. Black oxide of manganese was mined and employed in the making of chloroform. Other medically valuable products of Southern mines included alum, lime, and Epsom salts. Potassium sulfate, a byproduct of the manufacture of saltpeter (a vital constituent of gunpowder), was salvaged for medicinal use. Citizens of Columbia, South Carolina, delivered silver cups and plates to the army's local drug-manufacturing facility to be broken up and used in the production of silver nitrate. Dried Spanish flies (*Cantharis vesicatoria*), used commonly at the time as a blistering agent, could not be imported reliably, so citizens were asked to collect potato flies (*Cantharis vittata*) as a substitute; a "liberal price per pound" was offered for the dried insect. In at least one army drug manufacturing facility, animal bones and horns were processed into ammonia.[21]

Processing of Raw Materials

When gathered resources could not be used directly as medicines, they were typically sent to army drug manufactories, called medical laboratories, for processing. Such facilities not only prepared indigenous remedies but were "engaged . . . in the manufacture of medicines heretofore universally procured from abroad." Grinding the dried plants, usually the first step of processing the indigenous remedies, was carried out in the laboratories or by outside contractors. Further steps produced relatively concentrated formulations whose purpose, according to Prioleau, was to "retain the full properties of the plant at the same time taking up as little room in the Regimental [medicine] Chest and the Patients stomach as possible." Ethyl alcohol, needed for preparing tinctures, was not always available, so one purveyor substituted whiskey in its place.[22]

Medical officials also considered it desirable to isolate the active components of plants and prepare them as relatively pure formulations; this would facilitate the standardization of doses and the evaluation of clinical effectiveness. The ability to prepare isolates was not common in the

Confederate laboratories, especially among workers who were unfamiliar with the plants and lacked an easy way to determine which of their numerous parts produced the desired effects. Medical Purveyor Chisolm suggested hiring European scientists to assist with the chemical aspects of preparing the isolates, and Medical Purveyor Prioleau had local chemists attempting to isolate the active component of Georgia bark.[23]

Outfitting the laboratories was no easy matter. When apparatus could not be purchased locally, it might be obtained from other sources. The medical laboratory at Lincolnton, North Carolina, for example, purchased equipment from the North Carolina Military Institute in Charlotte. Other items for the Lincolnton facility—leaden chambers for the production of sulfuric acid, for instance—were fabricated with the help of personnel from the Tredegar Iron Works in Richmond and the Confederate Navy yard in Charlotte. The director of one medical laboratory requested approval to seize an "iron screw & its appurtenances," needed for the preparation of castor oil, from a local individual who had refused to sell, rent, or lend him the equipment. The Macon laboratory was unable to obtain the vacuum apparatus necessary to produce high-quality drug concentrates, and the extracts it produced, according to a medical inspector, were consequently "unfit for issue." Glass containers for the packaging of liquid medicines were in short supply because of the blockade, so medical purveyors purchased bottles of all sizes from citizens.[24]

Because the whiskey purchased by the medical department was expensive and sometimes "vile," Surgeon General Moore ordered medical purveyors to buy existing distilleries or build new ones so that operations could be within their control. A few such government-owned distilleries were functioning by the end of the war. Officials in Georgia, North Carolina, and Virginia, contending that grain should feed soldiers and the poor rather than be made into spirits, opposed having distilleries—even those operated by or contracting with the Confederate medical department—in their states. The Confederate Congress overruled that objection by authorizing the surgeon general and commissary general to establish distilleries or to contract for the manufacture of whiskey or other liquors.[25]

Intellectual Resources

The effort to turn Southern resources into medicines would have gone nowhere if not for the personnel of the medical laboratories, which were usually directed by medical purveyors. According to Porcher, many of the medical department's most competent clinicians became medical purveyors or ended up in other "high cathedral places." Expert practitioners or not, medical purveyors were not necessarily knowledgeable about large-scale drug production, so it was necessary to staff the facilities with men who had relevant scientific or technical expertise, if not actual experience making medicines. The Lincolnton laboratory, for example, was directed by Surgeon-in-Charge Aaron Snowden Piggot, a physician whose primary interests were geology, metallurgy, mining, and chemistry. Piggot was specially recruited by the medical department and given considerable freedom to establish a laboratory at a site of his choosing. His expertise served him in selecting a location that had a source of water power to operate the laboratory machinery and yet was conveniently close to fields where medicinal plants could be cultivated and to deposits of minerals needed to produce sulfuric acid. He was also knowledgeable enough to direct the construction of laboratory apparatus.[26]

Other highly skilled laboratory personnel included physicians Joseph LeConte and St. Julien Ravenel and educator-minister James Woodrow, who were expert in chemistry and conducted drug manufacturing operations at the Columbia laboratory. Physician-naturalist F. J. B. Rohmer and physician-chemist Charles O. Curtman oversaw laboratory operations at Mobile, Alabama, and Arkadelphia, Arkansas, respectively. Pharmacist-botanist Charles Mohr helped in the analysis and production of drugs at the medical laboratory in Mobile.[27]

Surgeon General Moore described the personnel of purveying depots, laboratories, and distilleries as "in a great measure expert chemists, druggists, and distillers, and men of professional skill, whose services are absolutely indispensable for the manufacture of medicines . . . and alcoholic stimulants." Many of the skilled workers were civilians, and protecting them from conscription, especially late in the war, was a serious concern of Moore and the directors of his manufacturing facilities. The laboratories' other personnel included clerks, couriers, guards, packers, porters, construction workers, and "workwomen."[28]

Virtues of Southern Medicines

Surgeons took awhile to get used to the idea of using indigenous medicines. Such items appeared in only about a tenth of some 260 requisitions filled by Medical Purveyor Prioleau in Macon between September 1862 and July 1863, with the largest orders for the items coming from other medical purveyors. In May 1864, the surgeon general again urged surgeons to employ indigenous remedies "in view of their intrinsic value and economy to the Government, and also the impracticability of procuring sufficient supplies of medicines from abroad." By late 1864, the majority of requisitions received at the Macon depot contained requests for indigenous preparations. This trend may have indicated a gradual acceptance among surgeons of the remedies' usefulness. It might also have reflected a realization that it was better to specify some preferred indigenous preparations than to have a medical purveyor send whatever he thought might suffice as substitutes for unavailable standard drugs.[29]

Among the most frequently ordered indigenous remedies were preparations of boneset, bloodroot, sumach, and Georgia bark. Probably the most commonly issued plant-based remedy was a tonic and antimalarial mixture variously known as compound tincture of indigenous barks, "old indig[enous]," medicated whiskey, and Moore's tincture. "From some cause, not difficult to understand," quipped a surgeon, "the patients all approved highly" of this concoction of whiskey in which the barks of dogwood, willow, and tulip tree had been soaked.[30]

The pharmaceutical quality and clinical effectiveness of the Southern-made medicines are best characterized as uneven. The products were described as ranging from unusable and "not surpassingly excellent" to comparable in "neatness of preparation" to "the best English and French preparations of similar character." The indigenous preparations produced some symptomatic benefit — a vindication of Moore's impression that they would prove useful — but, on the whole, were not considered as effective as the standard agents they replaced. One surgeon stated that the use of indigenous remedies disproved the belief of some physicians that the plants of a region could eradicate the illnesses peculiar to that region. "We have but little more than indigenous barks and roots with which to treat the numerous forms of disease," lamented another medical officer, no doubt wishing he had the full array of standard drugs at his disposal.[31]

By today's criteria, many standard allopathic drugs of the time were ineffective or unacceptably toxic, so the clinical benefit of producing them in the South may be best considered for the ones whose good points clearly overbalanced the bad. Quinine was unquestionably a valuable drug, at least when used to prevent or treat malaria, but it was not produced at all in the South, and the Confederates never found a substitute—not even Georgia bark—that was its equal. Other undoubtedly beneficial drugs were the opiates and the anesthetics chloroform and ether. The yield from Southern cultivation of opium poppies was small. Chloroform and ether were manufactured in the medical laboratories, but the amounts produced have not been determined. The Southern-made anesthetics, if adequate in quality, helped soldiers and eased the burden of medical purveyors hard-pressed to find the imported items in large quantities. The laboratories did manage to produce a few standard medicines in amounts large enough to remove the need for medical purveyors to purchase them on the open market at exorbitant prices.[32]

It has been suggested that drug shortages actually protected Southern soldiers from the more toxic standard medications, such as the mercurial compounds. Quinine, opiates, chloroform, and ether could also be in short supply, however, and their scarcity forced troops to endure malaria and pain. Moreover, among the standard medicines supplied in large quantities by the laboratories were calomel (mild chloride of mercury), mercury pills, and mercury ointment, so troops were not spared the adverse effects of those preparations. And while it is commonly belied that plant-based medicines are fairly benign, some can be quite harmful, and it is uncertain whether the indigenous remedies were, on the whole, less dangerous than the medicines they replaced. All in all, it is probably safe to say that Confederate soldiers were worse off because of drug shortages and that some of their suffering was mitigated by the efforts of the medical department to manufacture scarce drugs or provide substitutes for them.[33]

Conclusion

The Confederate Army's effort to make its own drugs—the only reasonable response to anticipated and real shortages during a prolonged conflict—was managed ably and encompassed a wide array of natural and intellectual resources. It is difficult with available records to assess the effect of Southern drug production in terms of lives saved or suffering allayed. What is certain is that a hard-working and imaginative group of medical officers and civilians did its part to help reduce the suffering of Southern soldiers and increase the fighting efficiency of the Confederate Army.

Abbreviations

OR: *The War of the Rebellion: A Compilation of the Official Records of the Union and Confederate Armies.* Washington: Government Printing Office, 1880-1901.

NARA: National Archives and Records Administration, Washington, D.C.

CRMD: Record Group 109 (War Department Collection of Confederate Records), ch. 6 (Medical Department), NARA.

JJC: Letter Book of Dr. J. J. Chisolm, Medical Purveyor, C.S.A., Columbia, S.C., May 24 to November 14, 1862, Wessels Library, Newberry College, Newberry, S.C. (transcribed by F. Terry Hambrecht).

ASP: Maj. A. Snowden Piggot Papers, Record Group 109, NARA.

Notes

1. Descriptions of Confederate successes in supplying ordnance include Frank E. Vandiver, *Ploughshares into Swords: Josiah Gorgas and Confederate Ordnance* (College Station: Texas A&M University Press, 1994) and C. L. Bragg, Charles D. Ross, Gordon A. Blaker, Stephanie A. T. Jacobe, and Theodore P. Savas, *Never for Want of Powder: The Confederate Powder Works in Augusta, Georgia* (Columbia: University of South Carolina Press, 2007).

2. War Department, *Regulations for the Army of the Confederate States, 1862* (Richmond: J. W. Randolph, 1862), 244-57; John M. Maisch, "Report on the Drug Market," *Proceedings of the American Pharmaceutical Association* 12 (1864): 187-200.

3. S. P. Moore to John C. Breckinridge, 9 Feb. 1865, *OR*, ser. 4, vol. 3, pp. 1073-76; S. P. Moore, Circular, 2 Apr. 1862, *OR*, ser. 4, vol. 1, p. 1041.

4. Alex Berman, "A Striving for Scientific Respectability: Some American Botanics and the Nineteenth-Century Plant Materia Medica," *Bulletin of the History of Medicine* 30 (January-February 1956): 7-31; Dan King, *Quackery Unmasked: Or a Consideration of the Most Prominent Empirical Schemes of the Present Time, with an Enumeration of Some of the Causes Which Contribute to Their Support* (Boston: David Clapp, 1858).

5. Samuel Preston Moore, "Address of the President of the Association of Medical Officers of the Confederate States Army and Navy," *Southern Practitioner* 31 (October 1909): 491-98. The purpose of the *USP* was to standardize the nomenclature and preparations of "substances which possess medicinal power...the utility of which is most fully established and best understood." The *USP*'s primary list included "articles which might be considered of standard character," whereas its secondary list included "substances as were deemed of secondary

or doubtful efficacy" and articles, particularly new ones, for which further investigation was warranted. *The Pharmacopoeia of the United States of America* (Boston: Wells and Lilly, 1820). The *USP* classification scheme continued in subsequent editions, and its listings at the onset of the Civil War were included in George B. Wood and Franklin Bache, *The Dispensatory of the United States of America* (Philadelphia: J. B. Lippincott, 1858). Joseph Carson, *Synopsis of the Course of Lectures in Materia Medica and Pharmacy, Delivered on the University of Pennsylvania* (Philadelphia: Blanchard and Lea, 1855); John G. Westmoreland, *A Syllabus of Lectures on Materia Medica and Therapeutics, Delivered in the Atlanta Medical College* (Atlanta: G. P. Eddy, 1857); Henry R. Frost, *Outlines of a Course of Lectures on the Materia Medica, Designed for the Use of Students, Delivered at the Medical College of the State of South Carolina*, 5th ed. (Charleston: James and Williams, 1858).

6.   Samuel E. Lewis, "Samuel Preston Moore, M.D., Surgeon General of the Confederate States," *Southern Practitioner* 23 (1901): 381-86.

7.   *General Directions for Collecting and Drying Medicinal Substances of the Vegetable Kingdom* (Richmond: Surgeon General's Office, 1862); S. P. Moore, Circular, 2 Apr. 1862, *OR*, ser. 4, vol. 1, p. 1041.

8.   S. P. Moore to T. H. Williams, 22 Jul. 1862, *OR*, ser. 4, vol. 2, pp. 13-14; W. H. Prioleau to James Stewart, 12 Aug. 1862, microfilm M346, roll 983, NARA.

9.   Mary Elizabeth Massey, *Ersatz in the Confederacy* (Columbia: University of South Carolina Press, 1993), 119; Jonathan M. Townsend, "Francis Peyre Porcher, M.D.," *Annals of Medical History* 1 (third series, 1939): 177-88; Norman H. Franke, *Pharmaceutical Conditions and Drug Supply in the Confederacy* (Madison: American Institute of the History of Pharmacy, 1955), 36.

10. Adjutant and Inspector General's Office, Special Orders no. 56, para. 5, 11 Mar. 1862; F. Peyre Porcher to Virginia Porcher, 15 Mar. 1862, Letters (1855-1862) of Francis Peyre Porcher, Medical University of South Carolina Library, Charleston; F. P. Porcher, "Resources of the Southern Fields and Forests," *De Bow's Review* 6 (new series, August 1861): 105-31.

11. S. P. Moore, Addendum to Adjutant and Inspector General's Office, Special Orders no. 121, para. 17, 27 May 1862, microfilm M267, roll 378, NARA; Moore, "Address of the President"; S. P. Moore to W. H. Prioleau, 16 Sep. 1862, CRMD, vol. 566; S. P. Moore to F. Peyre Porcher, 10 Jun. 1862, Wickham Family Papers, 1766-1955, Virginia Historical Society, Richmond; Porcher, "Resources" (1861); W. H. Prioleau to E. W. Johns, 15 Jul. 1862, CRMD, vol. 572.

12. Francis Peyre Porcher, *Resources of the Southern Fields and Forests, Medical,*

Economical, and Agricultural (Charleston: Evans & Cogswell, 1863); Evans & Cogswell to S. P. Moore, Invoice, 18 Mar. 1862, microfilm M346, roll 288, NARA. The range of topics covered in Porcher's book contributed to its being hailed as "without a doubt the most really valuable work which has been given to the public since the beginning of the war." "Resources of the Southern Fields and Forests," *Daily Dispatch* (Richmond), 16 April 1863, 2.

13. *Standard Supply Table of the Indigenous Remedies for Field Service and the Sick in General Hospitals* (Richmond: Surgeon General's Office, 1863); Samuel Preston Moore to W. H. Prioleau, 23 Apr. 1863, CRMD, vol. 740, pt. 1; S. P. Moore to W. H. Prioleau, 16 Feb. 1864, CRMD, vol. 741, pt. 1; S. P. Moore, Circular, 16 Apr. 1863, CRMD, vol. 740, pt. 1.

14. Guy R. Hasegawa and F. Terry Hambrecht, "The Confederate Medical Laboratories," *Southern Medical Journal* 96 (December 2003): 1221-30; Abstracts, CRMD, vol. 621; S. P. Moore to W. H. Prioleau, 16 Sep. 1862, CRMD, vol. 566.

15. Wood and Bache, *Dispensatory.* The regulations for the medical department also remained on the standard supply table, while textbooks on anatomy, chemistry, surgery, and other topics were stricken from the list. S. P. Moore to Medical Directors of Hospitals, 10 Mar. 1864, CRMD, vol. 135. J. J. Chisolm to E. W. Johns, 2 Oct. 1862, JJC; James Stewart to W. H. Prioleau, 29 Jul. 1862, microfilm M346, roll 983, NARA. The number of copies of the *USD* available to Confederate surgeons has not been determined. Reproducing it in the South should have been a relatively simple matter, compared with having Porcher prepare an entirely new work.

16. Francis P. Porcher, "Report on the Indigenous Medicinal Plants of South Carolina," *Transactions of the American Medical Association* 2 (1849): 667-862; Joseph Jones, "Indigenous Remedies of the Southern Confederacy Which May Be Employed in the Treatment of Malarial Fever," *Southern Medical and Surgical Journal* 17 (September, October 1861): 673-718, 753-87; Peterfield Trent, "Intermittent Fever Treated by Decoction of Gossypium herbaceum, or Cotton-Seed," *Charleston Medical Journal and Review* 9 (1854): 97-98; H. A. Ramsay, "Cotton Seed in Intermittent Fever," *Nashville Medical Journal* 1 (1854): 150-51; H. R. Frost, "Cotton Seed (Gossypium Herbaceum) as an Antiperiodic in Intermittent Fever," *Charleston Medical Journal and Review* 5 (1850): 416; Wood and Bache, *Dispensatory*, 388; Stiles Kennedy, "Turpentine as a Remedial Agent," *Medical and Surgical Reporter* 16 (1 June 1867): 458-59; "On the External Application of Oil of Turpentine as a Substitute for Quinine in Intermittent

Southern Resources, Southern Medicines 123

Fever, with Reports of Cases," *Confederate States Medical and Surgical Journal* 1 (January 1864): 7-8; S. P. Moore to N. S. Crowell, 18 Sep. 1863, CRMD, vol. 135.

17. Berman, "Striving"; *Standard Supply Table of Indigenous Remedies*; James Stewart to William H. Prioleau, 5 Aug. 1862, microfilm M346, roll 983, NARA; George W. Sites to George Scarborough Barnsley, 5 Jun. 1863, In *Records of Ante-Bellum Southern Plantations from the Revolution through the Civil War* (microfilm), ser. J, pt. 4, reel 43, ed. Kenneth M. Stampp (Bethesda: University Publications of America, n.d.).

18. S. P. Moore to W. H. Prioleau, 16 Sep. 1862, CRMD, vol. 566; Staff of the Southern Reform Medical College, *Southern Medical Reformer & Review* 9 (March 1859); W. H. Prioleau to S. P. Moore, 24 Sep. 1862, CRMD, vol. 572; W. T. Park, Notice, *Savannah Republican*, 3 October 1862, 2; M. S. Thomson to W. H. Prioleau, 10 Sep. 1862, microfilm M346, reel 1024 (file for Thompson [sic]), NARA. Thomson was also the mayor of Macon from 1860 to 1862.

19. S. P. Moore, Circular, 27 May 1863, *OR*, ser. 4, vol. 2, p. 569; J. J. Chisolm to E. W. Johns, 3 Jul. 1862, JJC; J. J. Chisolm to E. W. Johns, 9 Jun. 1862, JJC; W. H. Prioleau to Revd. Mr. Leckie, 19 Jun. 1862, CRMD, vol. 572; W. H. Prioleau to E. W. Johns, 6 Aug. 1862, CRMD, vol. 572.

20. Samuel Preston Moore, Circular, 19 Mar. 1863, *OR*, ser. 4, vol. 2, p. 442; James T. Johnson to A. S. Piggot, 13 Aug. 1863, ASP; T. S. Beckwith Jr. to A. S. Piggot, 5 May 1863, ASP; S. P. Moore to R. Potts, 26 Oct. 1863, CRMD, vol. 740, pt. 2; W. H. Prioleau to S. P. Moore, 21 Sep. 1862, CRMD, vol. 572.

21. William Gesner to A. S. Piggot, 13 Jul. 1863, ASP; Samuel Grose to A. S. Piggot, 25 Nov. 1863, ASP; George S. Blackie to S. P. Moore, 10 Jul. 1863, CRMD, vol. 750; L. N. Dunham, Contract, 29 Sep. 1863, ASP; William Tiddy, Contract, 1 Dec 1863, ASP; E. W. Johns to A. Snowden Piggot, 20 Nov. 1862, ASP; George S. Blackie to S. P. Moore, 27 Jun. 1863, CRMD, vol. 750; Robert Gustafson, "A Study of the Life of James Woodrow Emphasizing His Theological and Scientific View as They Relate to the Evolution Controversy" (Ph.D. diss., Union Theological Seminary, 1964), 98-99; Harriott Horry Rutledge Ravenel, "Memoir of Harriott Horry Rutledge Ravenel," in *South Carolina Women in the Confederacy*, vol. 1, ed. Mrs. Thomas Taylor and Sallie Enders Conner (Columbia: State Company, 1903), 322; S. P. Moore to W. H. Prioleau, 23 Apr. 1863, CRMD, vol. 740, pt. 1; James T. Johnson, Advertisement, *Western Democrat* [Charlotte], 26 May 1863; Joseph LeConte to A. S. Piggot, 28 Sep. 1863, ASP.

22. Hasegawa and Hambrecht, "Confederate Medical Laboratories"; S. P. Moore to John C. Breckinridge, 9 Feb. 1865, *OR*, ser. 4, vol. 3, pp. 1073-76; W. H. Prioleau

to S. P. Moore, 23 Dec. 1862, CRMD, vol. 627; J. J. Chisolm to E. W. Johns, 2 Oct. 1862, JJC.

23.   J. J. Chisolm to E. W. Johns, 4 Aug. 1862, JJC; W. H. Prioleau to S. P. Moore, 27 Apr. 1863, CRMD, vol. 627.

24.   W. J. Hayes to A. S. Piggot, 7 Feb. 1865, ASP; A. Snowden Piggot to S. P. Moore, 10 Jul 1863, ASP; A. Snowden Piggot to S. R. Mallory, 21 Oct. 1863, ASP; W. R. Johnston to Howard Smith, 18 May 1864, microfilm M331, roll 142, NARA; E. N. Covey, Extracts from Inspection Report, 9 Jul. 1864, CRMD, vol. 628; Joseph Jacobs, "Some of the Drug Conditions during the War Between the States, 1861-1865," *Proceedings of the American Pharmaceutical Association* 46 (1898): 192-213; M. Howard, Advertisement, *Western Democrat* [Charlotte], 22 July 1862, 3.

25.   J. J. Chisolm to J. C. Miller, 28 Mar. 1862, JJC; S. P. Moore to W. H. Prioleau, 11 Dec. 1863, CRMD, vol. 740, pt. 2; S. P. Moore to W. H. Prioleau, 18 Mar. 1863, CRMD, vol. 740, pt. 1; S. P. Moore to John C. Breckinridge, 9 Feb. 1865, *OR*, ser. 4, vol. 3, pp. 1073-76; S. P. Moore to W. H. Prioleau, 4 May 1864, CRMD, vol. 628; Z. B. Vance to James A. Seddon, 31 Dec. 1863, and S. P. Moore, endorsement, 5 Jan. 1864, *OR*, ser. 4, vol. 2, pp. 1072-73; George Davis to James A. Seddon, with enclosures, 30 Nov. 1864, *OR*, ser. 4, vol. 3, pp. 875-80; An act to authorize the manufacture of spirituous liquors for the use of the Army and hospitals, 14 Jun. 1864, *OR*, ser. 4, vol. 3, pp. 481-82.

26.   F. Peyre Porcher, "Suggestions Made to the Medical Department. Modifications of Treatment Required in the Management of the Confederate Soldier, Dependent upon His Peculiar Moral and Physical Condition; with a Reference to Certain Points in Practice," *Southern Medical and Surgical Journal* 1 (series 3, September 1866): 248-86; Guy R. Hasegawa, "'Absurd Prejudice': A. Snowden Piggot and the Confederate Medical Laboratory at Lincolnton," *North Carolina Historical Review* 81 (July 2004): 313-34.

27.   Joseph LeConte to A. S. Piggot, 28 Sep. 1863, ASP; Ravenel, "Memoir," 320; J. W. Flinn, "Sketch Published in The State, of Columbia, and The News and Courier, of Charleston, January 18, 1907," In *Dr. James Woodrow as Seen by His Friends*, ed. Marion W. Woodrow (Columbia: R. L. Bryan, 1909), 4-32; T. Peyton Norville. "F. J. B. Rohmer, M.D.," In *Twice Remembered: Moments in the History of Spring Hill College*, ed. Charles J. Boyle (Mobile: Friends of Spring Hill College Library, 1993), 81-83; Samuel Worcester Butler, *The Medical Register and Directory of the United States* (Philadelphia: Office of the Medical and Surgical Reporter, 1874), 403; "Karl Theodor Mohr: Eine Biographische Skizze," *Pharmaceutische Rundschau* 5 (February 1887): 4-12.

28.   S. P. Moore to John C. Breckinridge, 9 Feb. 1865, *OR*, ser. 4, vol. 3, pp. 1073-76; S. P. Moore to Adjutant & Inspector General, 11 Feb. 1865, letter 1865C277, microfilm M474, roll 155, NARA; W. H. Prioleau, Payroll no. 1664, Nov. 1863, Record Group 109, ch. 2, entry 56, NARA.

29.   Requisitions, CRMD, vols. 567 and 571; Samuel Preston Moore to Medical Directors in the Field and Hospitals, Circular No. 8, 9 May 1864, *OR*, ser. 4, vol. 3, p. 402.

30.   Abstracts, CRMD, vol. 621; E. S. Gaillard, *The Medical and Surgical Lessons of the Late War* (Louisville: Louisville Journal Job Print, 1868): 9; S. P. Moore to W. H. Prioleau, 5 Dec. 1862, CRMD, vol. 739, pt. 2.

31.   Hasegawa and Hambrecht, "Confederate Medical Laboratories"; E. N. Covey, Extracts from Inspection Report, 9 Jul. 1864, CRMD, vol. 628; William H. Taylor, "Some Experiences of a Confederate Assistant Surgeon," *Transactions of the College of Physicians of Philadelphia* 28 (third series, 1906): 91-121; "Confederate Medicines," *Charleston Mercury*, 6 September 1864, 2; Gaillard, *Medical and Surgical Lessons*, 12-13; J. Crews Pelot to E. D. Eiland, 5 Sep. 1864, *OR*, ser. 2, vol. 7, pp. 773-74.

32.   Guy R. Hasegawa, "Quinine Substitutes in the Confederate Army," *Military Medicine* 172 (June 2007): 650-55; Moore, "Address of the President"; S. P. Moore to Richard Potts, 9 Jul. 1863, CRMD, vol. 740, pt. 2.

33.   James O. Breeden, "Medical Shortages and Confederate Medicine: A Retrospective Evaluation," *Southern Medical Journal* 86 (September 1993): 1040-48; S. P. Moore to Richard Potts, 9 Jul. 1863, CRMD, vol. 740, pt. 2; T. C. Hindman to S. Cooper, 19 Jun. 1863, *OR*, ser. 1, vol. 13, pp. 28-44; Abstracts, CRMD, vol. 621; Franke, *Pharmaceutical Conditions*, 38; Hasegawa, "Quinine Substitutes."

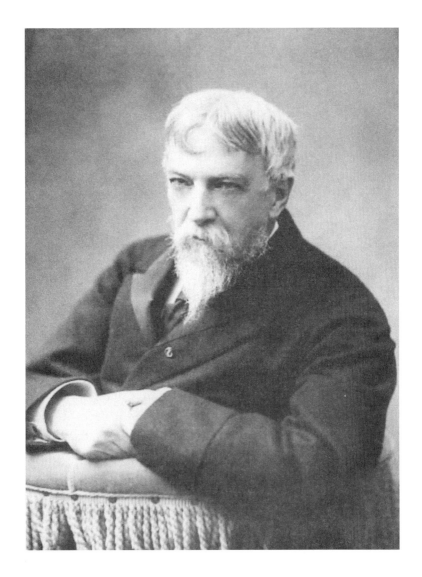

An original photograph of S. Weir Mitchell by Franz Meynen,
Artist & Photographer, 601 N. Marshall Street, Philadelphia,
Source: Author's collection

- 7 -

"The Firm"

Mitchell, Morehouse, and Keen and Civil War Neurology

D. J. Canale, M.D., F.A.C.S.

The American Civil War resulted in many new and original observations on the treatment of diseases and injuries resulting from gunshot wounds and exposure to infectious agents and the elements. In describing the challenges—and opportunities—that all wars provide, one historian declared, "Medicine is probably the only non-belligerent profession in which progress has been made as the direct result of war, and the challenge of war to the physician is perhaps greater than that to any other member of society." Silas Weir Mitchell—along with his coworkers George R. Morehouse and W. W. Keen—took advantage of the unique opportunities that the Civil War afforded for the study of diseases and injuries of the nervous system. Keen referred to the team of three as "The Firm," and one historian opined that "American neurology was cradled and developed in the army during the Civil War," largely due to the impetus of Mitchell and his colleagues.[1]

S. Weir Mitchell was born in Philadelphia in 1829. His father, John Kearsley Mitchell (1793-1858), was a prominent Philadelphia physician. In addition to his busy practice, the elder Mitchell held the chair of medicine at Jefferson Medical College. J. K. Mitchell also conducted chemical experiments that were observed with interest by the younger Mitchell. S. Weir Mitchell attended the University of Pennsylvania and later graduated from Philadelphia's Jefferson Medical College in 1850. While a student at Jefferson, he assisted in the laboratory of Robley Dunglison, considered the "Father of American physiology." Following graduation from medical school, he traveled to Europe where he studied under Claude Bernard, whose influence further kindled his interest in experimental physiology.

Mitchell found it necessary to return to Philadelphia after a year abroad to assist his father, whose health was failing. In addition to his private practice, Mitchell established a laboratory of experimental physiology, and by the late 1850's he had published several reports on his physiologic researches. He later collaborated with William Hammond on a series of experiments. Hammond, then an army surgeon, was granted a year's leave to work with Mitchell in Philadelphia. The friendship would subsequently have major implications on Mitchell's career early during the Civil War. Mitchell's experiments on snake venoms culminated in his important monograph *Researches upon the Venom of the Rattlesnake*, published in 1860. Medical historian W. Bruce Fye declared that Mitchell was already America's leading experimental physiologist in 1863 when he applied—unsuccessfully, as it turns out—for the chair of physiology at the University of Pennsylvania.[2]

At the outbreak of the Civil War, Mitchell was offered the position of brigade surgeon in the United States Army medical department, but he declined because he felt responsible for the care of his recently widowed mother. Additionally, he had assumed responsibility for his father's medical practice. As things turned out, this was a fortuitous decision for both Mitchell and the future of American neurology. Mitchell's interest in the physiology of the nervous system is evidenced by his correspondence with Charles Eduard Brown-Sequard as early as 1861 (Brown-Sequard is said to be the inspiration for Robert Louis Stevenson's "Dr. Jekyll and Mr. Hyde"). By 1862, Mitchell had been appointed a contract surgeon with the U. S. Army. His first assignment was to the Filbert Street Hospital in Philadelphia in October 1862, an account of which is given in his first novel, *In War Time*. As a contract surgeon, Mitchell would have been able to continue at least part time his own private medical practice and even his physiologic researches.[3]

It was at the Filbert Street Hospital where Mitchell first began to concentrate his interest in injuries and diseases of the nervous system arising from war injuries. Recognizing his special interest, other surgeons began referring nerve injuries to the instiution. As the case load increased, Mitchell recognized the unique opportunity afforded him in which he had charge of treating a large concentration of nerve injuries and other neurological disorders. At his suggestion, Mitchell's close friend William Hammond, then Surgeon General, arranged for the establishment of the first hospital in the United States devoted to injuries and diseases of the nervous system in May, 1863. This was the U.S. Army Hospital, Christian Street, Philadelphia.

Surgeon General Hammond requested that George Read Morehouse be assigned to the Christian Street Hospital to share the workload as Mitchell's assistant. Morehouse was also a graduate of Jefferson Medical College and worked with Mitchell prior to the war on a research project concerning reptilian physiology. Additionally, Mitchell requested the Surgeon General to free him and Morehouse of the usual time-consuming administrative duties inherent in military hospitals. Hammond agreed to this request, which allowed Mitchell and Morehouse to devote most of their time to their cases.[4]

Ironically, it was in May 1863 that Mitchell learned he was not elected to the chair of physiology, which he had sought at the University of Pennsylvania, despite having the overwhelming support of the medical community. One can speculate that had Mitchell won the appointment, the investigation of nerve injuries may have not gone to completion, and Mitchell may not have risen to be one of the founders of clinical neurology in America.

The third member of Mitchell's group was William Williams Keen. Keen also had helped Mitchell with his physiologic researches while a student at Jefferson Medical College in 1860. Keen was appointed assistant surgeon after the war commenced and served at the first battle of Bull Run in July 1861. This defeat of the Union Army was compounded by the total lack of organization of the U.S. medical corps in the field. Nevertheless, Keen was said to have served with distinction. Following the battle, Keen returned to Jefferson Medical College, where he received his M.D. in March 1862. Keen was fortunate to have been a private office student of Jacob M. DaCosta and later John Hill Brinton, who taught Keen many of his practical surgical skills. Brinton had a distinguished career as surgeon in the U.S. Army.[5]

Shortly afterwards, Keen was appointed acting assistant surgeon in the U.S. Army. After several assignments, including being present at the Second Battle of Bull Run in August 1862, Keen was assigned to the Satterlee Hospital in Philadelphia. In early 1863, at Mitchell's request, Keen was assigned to the Christian Street Hospital where he would live as resident surgeon. Mitchell's team was now complete with the addition of Keen, the only one of the three with battlefield experience.[6]

The patient load increased at the Christian Street Hospital to the extent that the patients, Mitchell, and his colleagues were moved to the newly constructed 400-bed United States Hospital for Injuries and Diseases of the Nervous System at Turner's Lane, Philadelphia. The hospital was built according to the pavilion style, which was recognized earlier as best suited to military purposes. This was the first hospital in America devoted primarily for the treatment of neurological injuries and disorders of the nervous system and served as the first neurological research center. There would be no shortage of referrals to this specialty hospital, in which one ward was for the study and treatment of disorders of the heart under the direction of Jacob M. DaCosta, Keen's former mentor.[7]

One cannot overestimate William Hammond's importance to this endeavor. Had Hammond not been selected as Surgeon General over the objections of Secretary of War Edwin M. Stanton, Mitchell and his coworkers might not have had the opportunity to study the effects of gunshot injuries to nerves. While one historian identified S. Weir Mitchell as the catalyst who formed the team, all of the men seemed to recognize the unique opportunity before them and worked tirelessly into the night or early morning hours several days a week. Mitchell and Morehouse would arrive early in the morning for brief rounds, attend to their private practice, then return in the late afternoon.[8]

The principal observations they made in studying nerve injuries—in addition to the direct consequences of gunshot wounds (pain, paralysis, and loss of sensation)—related to reflex paralysis, causalgia, malingering, and phantom limb syndrome.

Gunshot Wounds

The results of investigations arising from the team's work at the Christian Street and Turner's Lane Hospitals were given in the monograph *Gunshot Wounds and Other Injuries of Nerves*, published in Philadelphia in 1864. This extremely scarce monograph has been described as "one of the acknowledged classics of nineteenth-century American medicine." It is a testimony to the authors' industry that they could bring to publication their observations with the war still in progress. Mitchell, being familiar with the publi-

GUNSHOT WOUNDS

AND OTHER

INJURIES OF NERVES.

BY

S. WEIR MITCHELL, M.D.
GEORGE R. MOREHOUSE, M.D.
AND
WILLIAM W. KEEN, M.D.
ACTING ASSISTANT SURGEONS U.S.A.

IN CHARGE OF U.S.A. WARDS FOR DISEASES OF THE NERVOUS SYSTEM, TURNER'S LANE
HOSPITAL, PHILADELPHIA.

Title page of *Gunshot Wounds and Other Injuries of Nerves*, 1864
Source: Author's collection

cations of the clinical neurologist community in London and Paris, was aware that the observations in the monograph were entirely new.[9]

Indeed, Mitchell and his colleagues stated that "never before in medical history has there been collected for study and treatment so remarkable a series of nerve injuries." This small book is also recognized as a classic in the history of neurology. In a sense, it marks the dawn of clinical neurology in America, and soon after the end of the Civil War, schools of clinical neurology would come into being in Philadelphia and New York.[10]

The number of cases of gunshot wounds of the major nerves during the Civil War is not recorded. One can safely assume that the number was not small, as official records account for nearly 90,000 gunshot wounds to the upper extremity and an equal number to the lower extremity. In writing *Gunshot Wounds*, Mitchell and his colleagues drew from more than a hundred carefully documented cases. Of these, they chose forty-eight cases, which they characterized by their location (spinal cord, cranial nerves, major nerves in the upper extremity, etc.).[11]

Mitchell classified injuries to the nerve trunks as (1) direct injury (partial or complete) by a missile, (2) commotion from near passage of a missile, (3) contusion, as from a blow, (4) injury resulting from dislocation or from attempts at its reduction, (5) cicatrix pressure, or (6) extension of disease from wounded to healthy nerves.

Typical of the detailed case studies was that of a soldier wounded at Gettysburg:

Case 19—Jacob Bieswanger, age 39, boxmaker, enlisted August, 1861, Co. B, 75th Pennsylvania Vols. Healthy to date of wound. July 1, 1863, at Gettysburg, while capping his gun, he was shot from the rear, through the left shoulder. The ball entered on a level with the fifth dorsal vertebra, an inch to the left of its spine, and emerged one-quarter of an inch above the left clavicle, piercing the outer edge of the sterno-cleido mastoid muscle, two inches from the sterno-clavicular articulation. The arm fell, bleeding a good deal, and thus only he knew he was hit. Then he examined the arm, and found it devoid of motion and sensation. After walking a little way, he fell, fainting and unconscious. Reviving shortly after, he began to spit blood, and continued so to do for a few days, without further evil as regarded the lungs. He lay on the field and in field hospitals four days—dressings being applied on the fourth day only. No splints used then or later.

He could not say when the wound healed, but is sure the pain began at or about that time. It was a prickly feeling in the pectoral region, shoulder, arm, forearm, and hand, where it was worse. It is now scarcely perceptible. There was no burning.

Sensation improved from above downward, as the wound healed. About the end of the fourth month, the shoulder movements returned in part, but the fingers moved feebly more than a month previous to this date.[12]

Bieswanger arrived in the care of Mitchell and his team in early December 1863, about six months after he was wounded. They took precise measurements of his wrist, forearms, biceps, and other muscles and structures and noted significant atrophy due to the wound. They also took casts of the soldier's arms and shoulders and sent them as specimens to the fledgling Army medical museum, as they showed "excellently all these deformities." They followed with precise observations of Bieswanger's range of motion and extension and sensitivity to touch, pain, and temperature. The surgeons followed with unspecified treatments, noting that the soldier was discharged "greatly improved."[13]

Surgery for gunshot wounds of the extremities was directed at arresting hemorrhage and performing amputations for compound fractures which, if delayed, often resulted pyemia and death. Indeed, Mitchell and his team did not record any cases in which a gunshot wound of an extremity was explored with the intention of repairing the nerve. Conventional wisdom on surgically repairing nerves was mixed. Longmore—in his wartime *Treatise on Gunshot Wounds*—only suggested removal of foreign bodies lodged against major nerves in order to prevent possible later symptoms. However, Samuel D. Gross's *System of Surgery* noted the importance of approximating the ends of larger nerves with sutures, while his own (but shorter) *Manual of Military Surgery*—for use in the field—did not address repair of severed nerves. The popular American edition of Erichsen's *Surgery*—edited by John H. Brinton and said to have been issued early in the war to Union surgeons—suggested that restoration of function eventually occurred without surgical repair.[14]

It must be assumed that a severed nerve without other major injury to an extremity was an uncommon event and rarely if ever a surgical priority. In Mitchell's later major treatise on injuries of nerves, he described his own physiologic experiments on degeneration and regeneration of severed nerves. He experimented on suturing together the divided ends of nerves in animals. The results were conclusive in demonstrating that recovery of nerve function was much enhanced by reapproximating by suture the divided ends of nerves.[15]

Reflex Paralysis

The team's first report of reflex paralysis was the aptly titled *Reflex Paralysis*, issued March 10, 1864, by the Surgeon General's office as circular no. 6. This study originated from the U.S. General Hospital, Christian Street, Philadelphia. In this report, Mitchell, Morehouse, and Keen reported a series of seven cases "in which paralysis of a remote part or parts has been occasioned by a gunshot wound of some prominent nerve or of some part of the body which is richly supplied by nerve branches of secondary size and importance." They made a distinction between shock (with vasomotor collapse resulting from blood loss) and blast injuries. The team postulated that a similar shock affecting the vasomotor centers (the nerves and muscles that cause the blood vessels to constrict or dilate) of the spinal cord and brain stem might result in interruption of reflexes at remote nerve centers.[16]

The conclusions were drawn not from personal observations but rather from later recollections of injured soldiers. These soldiers were seen after they had been treated in other general hospitals and transferred at a later date to the care of Mitchell and his associates. Mitchell noted utmost care was exercised in obtaining a history from their patients and moreover, they were usually "possessed of at least some education, and often of considerable intelligence and power of observation." The authors noted that only seven cases of reflex paralysis were identified in over sixty nerve wounds studied up to that time and suggested that many cases were slight or transient and easily overlooked by busy surgeons in the battlefield. The wartime circular on reflex paralysis was reprinted in 1941 by the Historical Library, Yale University School of Medicine. In his introductory note, John F. Fulton described the circular as "one of the great milestones in the history of American neurology."[17]

Causalgia

Among the major consequences of major nerve injuries that Mitchell and his team observed among wounded soldiers was a disabilitating burning pain observed after a *partial* injury to a major nerve. The pain—at times unbearable for the sufferer—was described as "burning or as mustard red hot, or as a red-hot file rasping the skin." The onset of the pain was delayed for a short time after the injury. The pain most often involved the plam of the hand and fingers and the dorsum of the foot. The most effective treatment was the avoidance of air by keeping the affected part wet using a bottle of water and a sponge. Noises and vibrations could increase the pain. Eventually, the affected part exhibited increased temperature and glossy skin.[18]

The condition would later be termed "causalgia," the term first appearing in 1867 in Mitchell's paper "On Diseases of Nerves, Resulting from Injuries." The term was suggested to Mitchell by his friend Robley Dunglison and was derived from the Greek for "burning" and "pain." In the paper, Mitchell noted that in fifty wartime cases of partial nerve injuries, causalgia existed in different degrees in nineteen cases. He expanded on the treatment of symptoms resulting from nerve injuries including other neuralgias and chorea-like movements in addition to causalgia. In addition to wet dressings and avoidance of heat for causalgia patients, other treatments included morphine injections, opium plasters, Fowler's solution, leeching, and cupping. In cases of paralysis, active and passive exercises, massage, splinting, and electrical stimulation were found to be useful. The credit with first studying and defining the symptoms of causalgia belongs to Mitchell and his coworkers.[19]

Malingering

Historians have noted that malingering was a major problem during the American Civil War. Malingering—or feigned disability—is defined "as the willful fabrication of physical or emotional symptoms to avoid an unwanted duty." Keen and his associates published an important and comprehensive paper, "On Malingering, Especially in Regard to Simulation of Diseases of the Nervous System." Their observations were taken from numerous cases seen at the Christian Street and Turner's Lane Hospital.[20]

The motives of malingerers were to seek discharge (and perhaps reenlist to obtain an additional enlistment bounty) and especially to avoid strenuous work or hazardous duty. A wartime surgeon listed eight classes of feigned illness affecting all organ systems. Many of the feigned illnesses involved the nervous system. Those symptoms of feigned illness observed by Keen included lameness, anchylosis, epilepsy, paralysis, blindness, deafness, aphonia, and others. The surgeons developed a suspicion when the symptoms were unusual. A system of "espionage" was developed to have informants spy on those suspected of feigning an illness.

They also devised a number of tests to expose feigned illness. Some soldiers seeing one of their fellows get out of hard duty would resort to imitating the symptoms, while others would report the malingerer to the medical staff. Malingering was most often encountered in the general hospital, especially among the less educated. Chronic rheumatism was so frequently a feigned symptom that the War Department issued a general order in 1862 prohibiting discharges for rheumatism. These cases were best handled by confronting the individual in the presence of his fellow soldiers or assigning him to the dirtiest work in the hospital. Allowing malingerers to go unpunished was bad for morale. Transfer to the Invalid Corps or court martial was less often resorted to.[21]

Phantom Limbs

Mitchell—describing the wards at Turner's Lane Hospital—noted, "Here at one time were eighty epileptics, and every kind of nerve wound, palsies, chorea, stump disorders." The 253-bed South Street Hospital—referred to as the "Stump Hospital" by the soldiers—was filled with amputees in need of artificial limbs. While there was never a thorough study of the patients at this hospital, Mitchell and his associates nevertheless recorded the neurological complications of many amputees under their care.[22]

A remarkable article, published anonymously in *The Atlantic Monthly* in 1866, entitled "The Case of George Dedlow" brought the attention of the general public for the first time to disabling consequences of nerve injuries. S. Weir Mitchell was the author of this article, which described in detail the symptoms of both causalgia and phantom limb syndrome before either condition had been named in the medical literature. It elicited much interest of the public to the plight of the fictional assistant surgeon George Dedlow. This short story also illustrated many aspects of the medical department during the war.[23]

Mitchell is largely responsible for describing the neurological symptoms resulting from amputations. Mitchell estimated that 15,000 men lost an arm or leg in the war (Mitchell underestimated: Union medical records reveal there were nearly 30,000 amputations). His article "Phantom Limbs"—published in 1871—was the first comprehensive report on the condition. The symptoms were actually the result of a nerve injury (the severed nerve in the amputated limb). Mitchell noted that the "stump" is "liable to the most horrible neuralgias, and to certain curious spasmodic maladies." These symptoms were often noted to be influenced by changes in the weather. Mitchell noted that nearly every man who loses a limb "carries about with him a constant or inconstant phantom of the missing member, a sensory ghost."[24]

The sensation of the missing limb could come on immediately upon awakening from the anesthetic or within the following two weeks. Mitchell and his team observed that rarely was there awareness of the entire missing limb, but more often a hand or foot. Other symptoms arising in amputations were neuralgia with varying degrees of neuritic pain and involuntary muscle contractions, which Mitchell termed "chorea of stumps." The neuritis was treated locally with cold, leeches, and counterirritants. Intractable pain occasionally necessitated resection of the nerve ending more proximal in the stump.

The long hours and stress took its toll on Mitchell in 1864 when he "broke down." He took two months leave and went to Paris and London. Mitchell afterwards returned to Philadelphia and Turner's Lane Hospital and again took up his researches until the hospital closed in June 1865.

Postwar Years

Following the war, Weir Mitchell continued with his busy private practice. His reputation as a neurologist soon led to his limiting his practice to neurological diseases. He shared many ideas and interests with the great French neurologist Jean-Martin Charcot during this period. In 1868, he once again (and, again unsuccessfully) sought a chair of physiology, this time at Jefferson Medical College. In 1872 he published *Injuries of Nerves and Their Consequences*, an expansion of the original study together with the anatomy and physiology of peripheral nerves. He also enlarged the sections on causalgia and phantom limbs. A follow up of twenty of the original cases was made by his son, John Kearsley Mitchell, in "Remote Consequences of Injuries of Nerves" in 1895.[25]

Mitchell began to write short stories shortly after the end of the war, but it was about 1880 that he began a second literary career based largely on the Civil War. The death of his brother Edward Donaldson Mitchell—a medical cadet—from diphtheria caused him great sorrow. One historian commented, "We can only mark, we cannot measure the effect of the Civil War upon Dr. Mitchell ... therefore it is ... when we read his tales and poems, no matter what the subject ... every drop of ink is tinctured with blood of the Civil War."[26]

Mitchell's appointment to Philadelphia's Orthopedic Hospital in 1870 proved to be important to his career as a neurologist. Because of his influence, it later became the Orthopedic Hospital and Infirmary for Nervous Diseases. He served actively until 1902, when he was appointed as consultant. Much of his future studies and publications would stem from this institution. Many honors would come to him in later years, including election as president of the American Neurological Association in 1909. Mitchell died in 1914. Such were his accomplishments that one historian declared, "no one during the Civil War occupies the position of Silas Weir Mitchell." Mitchell and Hammond later were considered the fathers of American neurology.[27]

George Read Morehouse enjoyed a successful private practice in Philadelphia following the war. He was a fellow of the College of Physicians and on the consultant staff of the Orthopedic Hospital but made no further contributions to neurology. He died in 1905.[28]

In the years following the war, William Williams Keen became a very distinguished anatomist and surgeon. His career spanned the last quarter of the nineteenth century, referred to as the "Golden Age" of American surgery. His experiences in the hospital for nervous diseases undoubtedly influenced his later career as an America's pioneer neurosurgeon. He was an early advocate of Joseph Lister's principles of antiseptic surgery after hearing Lister's address in Philadelphia in 1876. In 1887 he was the first in this country to successfully remove a brain tumor after clinically localizing the lesion. The patient lived for thirty years following the tumor removal. The following year Keen became professor of surgery at Jefferson Medical College. Keen greatly encouraged the young Harvey Cushing in the early

1900s at the beginning of the era of modern neurological surgery. Among his many honors was his election as president of the American Surgical Association in 1899 and the American Medical Association in 1900. Keen, the last survivor of "The Firm," died in 1932."[29]

Notes

1. John F. Fulton, "Neurology and War," *Transactions and Studies of the College of Physicians*, 8 (1940): 157-65; Lawrence C. McHenry, *Garrison's History of Neurology* (Springfield, MA: Charles C. Thomas, 1969), 326-27.
2. S. Weir Mitchell, *Researches upon the Venom of the Rattlesnake* (Washington: Smithsonian, 1861); W. Bruce Fye, "S. Weir Mitchell, Philadelphia's 'Lost Physiologist,'" *Bulletin of the History of Medicine*, 57 (1983): 188-202.
3. Christopher G. Goetz and Michael J. Aminoff, "The Brown-Sequard and S. Weir Mitchell Letters," *Neurology*, 57 (2001): 2100-2104; S. Weir Mitchell, *In War Time* (Boston: Houghton Mifflin, 1885); Anna R. Burr, *Weir Mitchell: His Life and Letters* (New York, Duffield, 1929), 104; S. Weir Mitchell, "Some Personal Recollections of the Civil War," *Transactions of the College of Physicians of Philadelphia*, 27 (1905): 87-94.
4. S. Weir Mitchell, *Injuries of Nerves and Their Consequences* (Philadelphia: J. B. Lippincott, 1872), 2-9.
5. S. Weir Mitchell, George R. Morehouse, William W. Keen, *Gunshot Wounds and Other Injuries of Nerves* (Reprint with Biographical Introduction by Ira M. Rutkow, San Francisco: Norman, 1989), v-xiv.
6. James L. Stone, "W. W. Keen: America's Pioneer Neurological Surgeon," *Neurosurgery*, 17 (1985): 997-1010; Richard D. Walter, *S. Weir Mitchell, M. D.—Neurologist* (Springfield, MA: Charles C. Thomas, 1970).
7. Frank R. Freemon, "The First Neurological Research Center: Turner's Lane Hospital During the American Civil War," *Journal of the History of the Neurosciences*, 2 (1993): 135-42; Frank H. Taylor, *Philadelphia in the Civil War, 1861-1865* (Philadelphia: City of Philadelphia, 1913), 224-36.
8. William S. Middleton, "The Fielding H. Garrison Lecture: Turner's Lane Hospital," *Bulletin of the History of Medicine*, 40 (1966): 14-42.
9. S. Weir Mitchell, George R. Morehouse, William W. Keen, *Gunshot Wounds and Other Injuries of Nerves* (Philadelphia: J. B. Lippincott, 1864); Ira M. Rutkow, *The History of Surgery in the United States, 1775-1900* (San Francisco: Norman, 1988), 50.

10. Mitchell, Morehouse, and Keen, *Gunshot Wounds* (1864), 9-10.

11. *The Medical and Surgical History of the War of the Rebellion*, Surgical History, Volume II, Part III (Washington: Government Printing Office, 1883): 690.

12. Mitchell, Morehouse, and Keen, *Gunshot Wounds* (1864), 90.

13. Ibid, 91-92.

14. T. A. Longmore, *Treatise on Gunshot Wounds* (Philadelphia: J. B. Lippincott, 1862); Samuel D. Gross, *A System of Surgery*, Second Edition (Philadelphia: Blanchard and Lea, 1862), Vol. I: 665, Vol. II: 985; Samuel D. Gross, *A Manual of Military Surgery* (Philadelphia: J. B. Lippincott, 1861); John Erichsen, *The Science and Art of Surgery*, John H. Brinton, ed. (Philadelphia: Blanchard and Lea, 1854), 137-38.

15. Mitchell, *Injuries of Nerves*, 235-43.

16. S. Weir Mitchell, George R. Morehouse, William W. Keen, *Reflex Paralysis*, Circular No. 6 (Washington: Surgeon General's Office, 1864), p. 1.

17. Mitchell, Morehouse, and Keen, *Gunshot Wounds* (1864), 9-10; S. Weir Mitchell, George R. Morehouse, William W. Keen, *Reflex Paralysis*, Circular No. 6 (Reprint with Introduction by John F. Fulton, New Haven: Yale University School of Medicine, 1941). The confusion surrounding reflex paralysis is demonstrated by Haymaker's error in attributing the condition to wounds of the brain. Neurologist Russell DeJong pointed out that these cases of Mitchell's were probably not organic in origin and in fact had no neurophysiologic basis. In World Wars I and II, this phenomenon was not observed in cases of peripheral nerve injuries.

18. Mitchell, Morehouse, and Keen, *Gunshot Wounds* (1864), 101.

19. S. Weir Mitchell, "On Diseases of Nerves, Resulting from Injuries," in Austin Flint (ed.), *Contributions Relating to the Causation and Prevention of Disease, and to Camp Diseases* (New York: Hurd and Houghton, 1867), 412-68.

20. Frank R. Freemon, "Detecting Feigned Illness During the American Civil War," *Journal of the History of the Neurosciences*, 2 (1993): 239-41; R. Gregory Lande, *Madness, Malingering, and Malfeasance* (Washington: Brassey's, 2003); Wm. W. Keen, S. Weir Mitchell, and Geo. R. Morehouse, "On Malingering, Especially in Regard to Simulation of Diseases of the Nervous System," *American Journal of the Medical Sciences*, 48 (1864): 367-94.

21. Roberts Bartholow, *A Manual of Instructions for Enlisting and Discharging Soldiers* (Philadelphia: J. B. Lippincott, 1863).

22. Mitchell, "Personal Recollections," 87-94; Taylor, 224-36.

23. "The Case of George Dedlow," *The Atlantic Monthly*, July 1866, 1-11; D. J. Canale,

"Civil War Medicine from the Perspective of S. Weir Mitchell's 'The Case of George Dedlow,'" *Journal of the History of the Neurosciences*, 13 (2004): 7-21.

24. *Medical And Surgical History*, Surgical History, Vol. II, Part III: 877; S. Weir Mitchell, "Phantom Limbs," *Lippincott's Magazine of Popular Literature and Science*, 8 (1871): 563-69; Mitchell, *Injuries of Nerves*, p. 348.

25. Christopher G. Goetz, "Jean-Martin Charcot and Silas Weir Mitchell," *Neurology*, 48 (1997): 1128-32; Mitchell, *Injuries of Nerves*; John K. Mitchell, *Remote Consequences of Injuries of Nerves and their Treatment* (Philadelphia: Lea Brothers, 1895).

26. Owen Wister, "S. Weir Mitchell, Man of Letters," in *S. Weir Mitchell, 1828-1914, Memorial Addresses and Resolutions* (Philadelphia: College of Physicians of Philadelphia, 1914); D. J. Canale, "S. Weir Mitchell's Prose and Poetry on the American Civil War," *Journal of the History of the Neurosciences*, 13 (2004): 7-21; Ernest S. Earnest, *S. Weir Mitchell: Novelist and Physician* (Philadelphia: University of Pennsylvania, 1950), 92-124.

27. John F. Fulton, Medicine, Warfare, and History," *Journal of the American Medical Association*, 153 (1953): 482-88.

28. Howard A. Kelly and Walter L. Burrage, *Dictionary of American Medical Biography* (New York: D. Appleton, 1928).

29. William W. Keen, *The Surgical Operations on President Cleveland in 1893* (Philadelphia: J. B. Lippincott, 1928), 436-37; Stone, 997-1010.

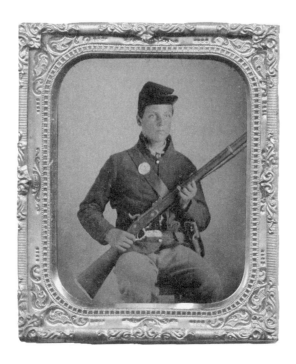

Tintype of an unidentified soldier. Recent research has
revealed that younger soldiers were at higher risk of
developing nervous ailments than their older comrades.
Source: Dennis M. Keesee Collection

- 8 -

"Haunted Minds"

The Impact of Combat Exposure on the Mental and Physical Health of Civil War Veterans

JUDITH ANDERSEN, PH.D.

In mid-January 1871 Nellie Kinsman Lang went before a judge in the City of Hastings, Dakota County, Minnesota, and testified to the physical and verbal abuse, neglect, and abandonment she and her two small daughters had suffered at the hands of her husband, twenty-nine-year-old Civil War veteran Frank Lang. In her testimony she recounted numerous episodes as evidence of the violent actions, explosive anger, and pent-up rage of the Civil War soldier she had married at the tender age of sixteen in 1865.

"My husband was continually cross and morose and violent in his disposition," she declared in the referee's report. On one occasion he exploded in violence because she had stayed at the neighbor's house too long. Another time she was helping him build a pigpen in the back yard when, "while holding a board for him to nail he said if I did not hold it still he would knock me over with the hatchet, he was very angry at this time I dropped the board and ran being in fear of him. . . . [He] threatened to strike me with the board and swore at me calling me vile and improper names."

On another occasion, "returning from his work in the evening and not finding supper ready inquired of me with anger why supper was not ready, I told him I had been washing hard all day which was the fact and I told him I would get it as soon as I could, whereupon he swore at me and ordered me to leave the house and took hold of me and attempted to hit me whereupon I went out and immediately returned, as I came in he was standing by the table . . . and taking from it a butcher knife swore I should not come drawing the butcher knife."[1]

Such violent outbursts were punctuated by prolonged periods of abandonment, such as the eight-month period in 1869 when Frank disappeared, returning around Thanksgiving, still "cross and morose." Nellie Lang had had enough. Her divorce papers demonstrate that Frank Lang's destructive actions had their intended effect: they destroyed his marriage. The court granted Nellie Kinsman Lang a divorce, and Frank never saw Nellie or his two daughters again.

Frank Lang was not just an average farm laborer; he had been an active-duty infantryman and hospital attendant in the Union Army during the American Civil War. His behaviors suggest an underlying psychological disorder that illustrates the lifelong impact of combat exposure on the mental and physical health of Civil War veterans.

Frank Lang (Franz Lange) was born in what later became Germany and came to the United States as a boy. Following in the footsteps of his friends and neighbors, Frank volunteered for infantry service in August of 1861, mustering into the ranks of Company K of the Seventh Michigan Infantry in the Union Army. For the next four years he served as a soldier and battlefield nurse, moving with the infantry and serving in makeshift hospitals through some of the most gruesome battles and marches on record. Of the ten most costly battles of the Civil War—based on wounded, killed, captured, and missing—the Seventh Michigan Infantry was involved in half of them (including Antietam, Chancellorsville, Gettysburg, Spotsylvania, and the Wilderness). Private Lang's regiment was witness to many other battles, including eight in which the loss was greater than 500 men, such as Savage's Station, Fredericksburg, Cold Harbor, and Petersburg.[2]

From military service records we know the places and battles in which Private Lang served, and from detailed descriptions of the battles and the hospitals we gain insight into how these war experiences marked his mind and shaped his future. For four years Private Lang lived and breathed combat. His war service was filled with exposures that we now know exacerbate the mental and physical effects of trauma: witnessing death and killing others, handling dead bodies, exposure to the elements (extreme heat and cold), malnutrition, exhaustion, and youth. According to Private Lang's declaration of age listed on his reenlistment papers he would have been about twenty-one years old at the beginning of his military service.[3]

The Makings of a Haunted Mind

As a field nurse/hospital attendant who was employed continuously, Private Lang was literally wading through blood and bodies, sorting the dead to find and rescue the living. Each new battle brought another set of horrors. Long after the firing of cannon would cease and the rescue began, the cries of the wounded could be heard—shrieks of pain, dying calls from brother to brother, or pleading calls for water or help. In a letter home to his fiancé, Private John Burrill of the Second New Hampshire Volunteers recounted the aftermath of the Battle of Gettysburg and his particular shock at rescuing a soldier, still alive with part of his head blown off:

> I went over the battlefield before the men were buried and they lay awful thick, I can assure you. I have been over other fields but never one like this. In one place I counted 16 in a spot no larger than your kitchen. It was a hard sight. They had turned black and swollen to twice their natural size . . . In going over, I saw one man who did not look like the rest. He was not black or swollen. He was alive. He could move his own hands a little. I went up to him and saw the top of his head was blown off. I gave him a little water—got some help—put him on a blanket and carried him to an old barn where he would get attention. He was about as hard a looking man as I ever saw and I have seen many. I have seen men torn in pieces in almost every shape and mind nothing of it, but not so with this one.[4]

The dead and wounded after Gettysburg were so abundant it took days to sort through the piles of black and swollen corpses and body parts strewn about. Day and night soldiers lay on the battlefield, trapped from rescue by enemy fire, their bodies flayed open by bullets. Private Lang witnessed death and handled the dying almost daily, likely tending to personal friends and neighbors among his fellow soldiers.

Exposure to extreme temperatures of heat and cold and overcrowded living quarters were common experiences for soldiers. The makeshift hospitals, such as those set up after the battle of Fredericksburg, in December 1863, were sometimes nothing more than flimsy tents where the ill and wounded lay on frozen ground, some without a blanket beneath them. The surgeons' stations were lined with piles of amputated limbs, reeking and decomposing, due to the great volume of surgeries and shortage of persons to clean up. The hospitals were often filled beyond capacity, but the wounded continually flooded in. As great numbers of wounded from Chancellorsville began to arrive at the closest hospital, there were not enough ambulance carts or medics to transport them. The wounded lay in the streets and on the wharf all night, exposed to heavy rain showers with no shelter. Records show that Private Lang served these dying and wounded soldiers in these uncomfortable settings throughout his entire service.[5]

Harsh living conditions were made worse by malnutrition and exhaustion. Union troops were provided with hardtack (sometimes full of weevils) and salted meat, cornmeal, coffee, and sometimes vegetable supplements. However, the rations were small and at times the meat was rancid, especially during marches where transportation of supplies was difficult. Some soldiers would eat through their three-day portion in a day and go hungry for some days afterward. The soldiers were required to march long distances (ten to twenty miles per day) carrying up to fifty pounds of gear. Combat, lack of sleep, long marches without food, and inadequate shoes (army shoes wore through in about twenty to thirty days of marching and were almost impossible to replace) and clothing (recruits were issued a single woolen uniform that was worn summer and winter, despite holes and soiling) added exponentially to physiological exhaustion.

What is clear from ancient and modern wars is that the combination of exhaustion, hunger, marching and fighting, all done at the mercy of the elements, is a recipe for psychiatric casualties. Private Lang's regiment was no stranger to hardship, experiencing a fifty percent casualty rate over the years of the war. Especially grueling conditions marked the long campaign that started in May 1864 at Barry's Hill and ended in the Siege of Petersburg. During this last push, the regiment crossed the Rapidan River and was swept into the terrible Battle of the Wilderness. Without rest they marched on to fight at Spotsylvania with great bloodshed. During a disastrous charge at Cold Harbor the Seventh Michigan suffered heavy loss. Battle after battle, the fighting continued for these soldiers through yet another year, culminating with the surrender of Confederate General Robert E. Lee on April 9, 1865, at Appomattox Court House. As a mark of dedication, Private Lang continued to serve despite contracting a hernia while traversing battleground trenches.

Mustering out of the Army in July 1865, Private Lang showed no visible

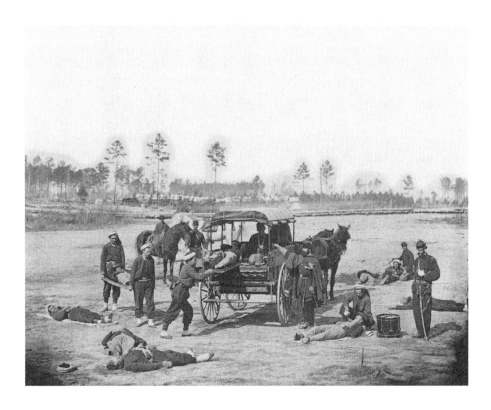

Removal of dead and wounded from the battlefield was one of the duties
that was required of Frank Lang as a field nurse/hospital attendant. This image
is of a Zouave ambulance crew demonstrating removal of wounded soldiers
from the field. *Source: Library of Congress*

wounds marking his experience, yet he carried memories that would haunt his mind and tear his family apart. In August 1865 he returned to a young bride he had married while on furlough months before. In 1866 she gave birth to a daughter. The threesome migrated from rural Michigan to Hastings, Minnesota, a bustling river town where Frank worked as a cooper. A second daughter was born in 1868. Less than three years later, in January 1871, illiterate and without property, Nellie Kinsman Lang filed for divorce. The divorce papers detailed Frank's explosive temper and extended periods of reclusiveness and neglect of his family. Before the court, Nellie recounted Frank's many bouts of physical violence, the long periods of abuse and neglect, and the wretched poverty, hunger, and destitution she and her children suffered. "My husband was continually cross & morose and violent in his disposition . . . [he] has frequently during our marriage threatened to strike me drawing his hand. . . . [he] never entered the house in good nature or pleasantly—[he] has said that when spring comes he would sell the house & lot and everything we had & leave me and the children and not leave me a chair to sit in."

Neighbors corroborated her account. The extremes of Frank Lang's behavior strongly suggest that he suffered enormous mental anguish directly rooted in his four-year experience as a Civil War soldier and field nurse. With no explanation for what he was feeling and no one to help him mentally process the great suffering he had witnessed, he could neither manage himself nor sustain a family. Nellie Kinsman Lang would very likely agree that his wartime experiences had changed him in profound and disturbing ways.[6]

Witnessing the carnage of war can leave permanent marks on one's mind and body. Examples of acute and posttraumatic stress reactions to the death and destruction of war have been noted throughout history and are not unique to the Civil War. However, the profound impact of the American Civil War on the culture and customs of the United States presents undeniable examples of this relationship. The sheer magnitude of carnage highlights the possibility of a link between mental and physical health reactions to war. An estimated 620,000 soldiers and upwards of 50,000 civilians died between 1861 and 1865 as battles raged across fields and farms, dividing towns and families alike. While anecdotal clues may suggest a link between war exposure and health, a systematic review—scientific, statistical, and clinical—of military and medical records of veterans from the Civil War demonstrates the impact of war trauma on both the mental and physical health of veterans over their entire lives.[7]

Battlefield Stress

The modern military and medical terms "Combat Stress Reaction" (CSR), "Acute Stress Disorder" (ASD), and "Posttraumatic Stress Disorder" (PTSD) are widely known and commonly used even in civilian rhetoric. These terms classify and categorize the reactions of individuals who have been exposed to trauma. The terms also make a distinction between immediate reactions, most likely experienced while on the battlefield (CSR, ASD), and delayed reactions (PTSD), symptoms that are displayed after the soldier is removed from battle (typically diagnosed if symptoms last longer than three months).[8]

Although these terms did not exist during the Civil War, examples of these reactions are common in both the medical and lay writings of the time. The gruesome war quickly overwhelmed the nation with the realities of desolation resulting from combat. Civilians who turned out to lunch and watch the First Battle of Bull Run quickly recognized that the war was no picnic. For years, battles were fought in the yards and barns of citizens. Homes and public buildings were converted to makeshift hospitals housing ill and wounded soldiers. Reminders of the conflict remained for years after the war ended. It is no wonder that within the medical community in North America the Civil War is associated with the initial recognition of how mental health is influenced by war trauma, both on and off the battlefield.[9]

Exposed to the mutilation and death of friends and comrades during direct combat, many soldiers respond with immediate and severe reactions. Physicians in the Civil War noted that stress reactions included paralysis, muteness, screaming, and weeping uncontrollably; some froze in place, unable to move, others fell to the ground and curled into the fetal position. In civilian psychiatry at that time, symptoms such as these were considered "hysterical" and were most often diagnosed among women exposed to intimate violence such as domestic abuse, rape, or incest. In the military, physicians initially categorized these profound reactions to war events as "Combat Hysteria." However, as the link between exposure to violence and death during war service and psychiatric symptoms became clearer, the categorization of reactions as "hysterical" seemed untenable.[10]

Studies show a dose-response relationship between the length and severity of combat exposure and the number of psychiatric casualties. Soldiers do not become accustomed to war over time; instead they have a breaking point. For example, ninety-eight percent of soldiers exposed to *continuous* combat on the beaches of Normandy in World War II became psychiatric causalities. Even the strongest soldier suffered a combat stress reaction after 200 to 240 days of intermittent combat in World War II, and the psychiatric casualty rate was in direct proportion to the severity of combat exposure. Combat stress reactions are now understood to be a natural display of the human revulsion to killing others and being under prolonged threat of death.[11]

Nostalgia

"Nostalgia" was a diagnosis given during the Civil War to active soldiers who were morose and weak during battle. This condition was thought to set in when soldiers were thrown into the tumult of war: viewing combat and experiencing the shockingly different environment of war (marching, illness, poor living conditions). It was noted that nostalgia, in severe cases, could lead to death because of the recruit's absolute hopelessness and that this was more likely to happen with young recruits. This diagnosis was used at an alarming rate during the first year of service. The U.S. Surgeon General later recommended the age of entry into service be increased, not over concern for the health of these recruits *per se* but to reduce the economic burden placed on society from hospitals flooded with homesick boys. Army Surgeon J. T. Calhoun suggested four factors for the prevalence of nostalgia: disease, discomfort, youthful volunteers who signed up for service in a hasty manner, and communications through letter-writing to loved ones at home. It was also hypothesized that this condition would be totally cured by returning the recruit to his home. Aside from illness, fatigue, and homesickness, there were other clues that combat marked the mind and body in dramatic ways. Even after returning home as victors, many veterans remained restless and unnerved. As history shows, the return to warm and embracing families, an outpouring of public gratitude in the form of parades and honors, as well as the heroic status of the Civil War veteran did not erase the haunting experiences of war.[12]

Posttraumatic Reactions to Civil War Combat

For some Civil War soldiers, reactions to combat continued—or sometimes surfaced for the first time—after the removal from the battlefield. Soldiers suffered from symptoms such as nightmares, flashbacks, anxiety, agitation, irritability, nervousness, unexplained headaches, and nausea. Several different terms arose to explain these mysterious mental health issues, such as "war neuroses" and "nervous disorders." With no observable organic origin, these symptoms were clustered under the umbrella diagnosis of nervous disease, or irregularities of the nervous system. Nervous disorders included mental health ailments such as paranoia, psychosis, hallucinations, illusions, insomnia, confusion, hysteria, memory problems, delusions, and violent behavior. This class of disease also included unexplained physical ailments of the nervous system (e.g., trouble with balance, incoordination, aphsia, paralysis, tremor, hyperaesthesia, vertigo, headaches, epilepsy, and memory loss). Although these nervous disorders were recognized by the medical community and diagnosed, they were not considered curable. These incurable symptoms presented military physicians with a perplexing problem for which two lines of thinking were explored: either an underlying "undiscovered" physical disease was causing these nervous symptoms or the soldier was of low moral character, cowardly, or decidedly malingering.[13]

The possibility of undiscovered disease as the root of nervous disorder was explored by noting clusters of related symptoms. One such cluster—functional disorders of the heart—was so commonly noted during the war years that it was termed "irritable heart" and "cardiac muscular exhaustion." Symptoms included irregular palpitations, unexplained racing heart, pain, and disorders of the heart in the absence of observable disease. These cardiac conditions were thought to be brought on by the anxieties and excitement of war as well as the overexertion of training, marching, and battle. Upon autopsies of soldiers who died from unrelated causes but had complained of the cardiac symptoms, physicians found that cardiac exhaustion and atrophy occurred only in *some* of the cases. This evidence indicated the root of these nervous conditions was not always of organic origin. Two commonly held explanations for this cluster of disorders were that the heart was thrown into irregularities by some other dysfunctional organ such as the stomach or liver, and that the soldier had been engaged in "vicious habits," which during the Civil War era were defined as the abuse of coffee, tea, or alcohol; masturbation and excessive sex.[14]

The mystery remained, however, in the lack of consistent functional or structural changes in the hearts of these deceased soldiers who had similar clusters of symptoms. At the time, war physicians and other military medical professionals did not account for the psychological impact of soldiers' experiences or make the link between mental health and physical disease.

Malingering

Unfortunately, throughout history, the medical community and the general public have repeatedly confused combat stress reactions with cowardice. Psychiatric reactions to terrifying combat events have often been associated with low moral character. This misconception is painfully obvious when reading the treatment recommendations for psychiatric war casualties published by prominent British psychiatrist Lewis Yealland during the WWI era. Treatments included threatening and punishing recruits who displayed "hysterical reactions." Although opposed by a few progressive psychiatrists recommending humane treatment, Yealland continued barbaric treatments, including the use of electric shock on the throats of soldiers who had become mute or paralyzed on the battlefield while simultaneously verbally shaming the soldier: "Remember, you must behave as the hero I expect you to be . . . .A man who has gone through so many battles should have better control of himself." Combat stress reactions have often been considered a weakness. Recruits who seek help for psychiatric reactions have been often categorized as malingerers, faking illness for monetary gain, or desiring to be removed from the war. Although malingering individuals constitute a portion of every war and are present in every medical setting, the take-home message is undeniable: A majority of individuals suffer some form of psychiatric casualty after witnessing *unremitting* war carnage; indeed, those that do not are rare and possibly personality disordered.[15]

Civil War Medical Records of Mental Health

In order to distinguish malingering soldiers from those with actual disease, the government developed a system of checks and balances. In 1862, the first Civil War-specific legislation regarding pensions was passed regarding the diagnosis and payment of veterans for wounds and illness directly related to military service. In order to avoid paying unnecessary pensions to soldiers feigning illness, pension boards developed detailed procedures for investigating claims. When a recruit filed a claim for a pension, a government examiner was assigned to review the military history and any hospitalizations of the veteran. If the wound or illness claimed was directly and obviously related to the war, the pension was assigned based on disability. If the wound or illness was not obviously related, the examiner would then interview both the claimant and other witnesses and collect sworn affidavits from family, friends, and "objective" townsfolk such as clergy, swearing that the veteran's condition was not present before the war and was as disabling as claimed.

Next, in order to prove the veracity of the claim the soldier was subject to a board of examining physicians who had to come to consensus about the claimant's condition and its relation to war service and the severity of the disability. Once a pension was granted, the veteran was reexamined by the pension board surgeons every alternate odd year to establish if the conditioned remained, was still pensionable, or needed an adjustment in severity rating. Despite the detailed instructions to pension board surgeons to diagnose only war-related disease, unrelated nervous disorders were commonly diagnosed. In 1890 the pension law was relaxed and allowed the diagnosis of disease and disability not related to war experience. However, multiple examinations by pension board surgeons were still required in order to establish and maintain the veracity of disease and disability claims.[16]

The Importance of Objective Evidence

We shudder at the story of Private Frank Lang, whose experiences during the war marked him — and his family — in a profound and terrible way. Reading the diaries of veterans, collections of small unit experiences, and letters between veterans and family members gives a clear picture of the deplorable conditions of war and the horrors that many experienced. This anecdotal evidence is important to help us understand the details of an almost unimaginable experience. However, the ability to make accurate predictions of the long-term consequences of traumatic war experience is predicated by examining objective evidence from many individuals and raises important clinical questions: were the experiences of the Civil

War enough to haunt the minds of soldiers for years to come in the form of posttraumatic stress? Is it possible that experiences that marked the minds of veterans were also related to the physical diseases they developed during their lives after the war?

Science and knowledge progress via the systematic examination of representative cases from a population of interest. While correlation does not imply causation, a systematic review of representative records allow us to be confident in our inferences about the relationships we find. Fortunately, a large number of Civil War military files (enlistment and discharge dates, age at enlistment, geographic location of company, and many other variables) and pension files (birth information, number of self-reported disease claims, physician diagnosed disease) were transcribed as part of the Early Indicators of Later Work Levels, Disease, and Death (EI) project. The EI project set forth to preserve the most comprehensive collection of Civil War records in a standardized format. The larger EI project randomly selected more than 300 companies of Union Army recruits (of 20,000 possible companies) from the descriptive roll books at the National Archives in Washington, D.C. The military service and pension files for 35,730 soldiers were then transcribed from handwritten records into computerized data files.[17]

Exploring Nervous Disease

In this large and detailed sample of Civil War medical records, multiple uniquely diagnosed nervous ailments and physical conditions (e.g. cardio-vascular and gastrointestinal ailments) were examined. As part of this project, physicians meticulously compared and coded conditions diagnosed in the Civil War era with modern disease categories. While Civil War era and modern medical diagnoses are not an exact match, there is actually significant overlap. The number of unique nervous ailments diagnosed in a veteran's record range from one to twenty-one with an average of 2.51. Soldiers in companies with the highest company mortality experienced a sixteen percent increased risk of developing multiple nervous ailments. Of great interest were the findings regarding wounded soldiers: veterans who were wounded during military service were less likely to ever develop signs of cardiovascular or gastrointestinal disease. However, these veterans had a sixty-four percent increased risk of developing nervous disease when compared to non-wounded men. An explanatory hypothesis for this dramatic increase in risk of developing a mental health diagnosis in the absence of physical disease may be physical hardiness. It is likely that soldiers who were physically tough enough to survive a battle wound in the unsanitary conditions of the Civil War were probably hardy individuals, and less likely to succumb to physical disease later in life. However, the psychological impact of being wounded often left a mark on even the sturdiest of soldiers.[18]

Soldiers who were younger when they first enlisted (younger than twenty years) were at a higher risk of developing a greater number of nervous ailments than their older peers. Soldiers who were eighteen or younger at enlistment had a thirty-eight percent increased risk of developing a number of unique nervous ailments compared to soldiers who were thirty years old at first enlistment. From the associations among these records it is apparent that witnessing death—especially at a young age—increased a soldier's risk of developing multiple nervous ailments across his lifespan.[19]

Lessons Learned

Exposure to the horrors of war comes with a price. Witnessing and participating in war marks a great number of soldiers with life-long mental and physical disease. Combat stress and posttraumatic stress reactions are not new phenomena associated with modern warfare. From a systematic review of Civil War military and medical records it is apparent that factors such as the age of the recruit at enlistment, company mortality, and being wounded increased the likelihood of mental health problems in Civil War soldiers. Modern experts in neurobiology posit a neurobiological explanation for the evidence that war exposure may have particular impact for young individuals. Brain regions that regulate emotion and nervous system activity are not fully developed until early adulthood. Adolescents younger than twenty years of age, in particular, may be at greatly increased risk of developing mental health problems due to immature neurological function.[20]

Unfortunately, the findings from this sample of military and medical records of Civil War veterans are not unlike the results we see from more modern samples. Physical and mental wounds remain life-long as a reminder of the exposure. We know this now, not just from anecdotal evidence, but from a representative sample of objective records. As a medical profession and society, we can begin to address these issues, not by blaming soldiers for weak characters and low moral fortitude, but by recognizing the link between war exposure and mental and physical disease and instituting early intervention programs to aid those in need.[21]

Frank Lang was young when he entered military service. He joined the Seventh Michigan Infantry, a regiment that experienced a fifty percent casualty rate across the years of his service. From the military and court records examined above we can see that Private Lang was at great risk of developing a nervous disease. He was haunted by his experiences on the battlefield as he was saving the lives of others. War exposure can influence not only the veteran, but the families of the soldiers. We can see from the records that not only was Private Lang marked by his war experiences, but that his young family suffered greatly upon his return. War, it seems, is an unceasing component of society. We must be vigilant in caring for those who face battle and to the families to which these soldiers return.

Notes

Data reviewed in this chapter was collected and summarized while supported by grant P01 AG 10120 from the National Institutes on Aging, Bethesda, MD, as a subgrant from the Center for Population Economics at the University of Chicago, Chicago, IL, and the National Bureau of Economics, Boston, Mass.

Roxane Cohen Silver, Ph.D., and JoAnn Prause, Ph.D., collaborated on the larger data analysis from which this chapter is drawn. Their help with data analysis and manuscript preparation was invaluable for the study published in the *Archives of General Psychiatry* and summarized in this chapter.

Michael J. Schroeder, Assistant Professor of History at Lebanon Valley College, Annville, PA., and his brother Tom Schroeder, provided excellent content and editorial contributions regarding Frank Lang and Nellie Kinsman Lang.

Thank you to Larry Lantinga, Ph.D., Vanessa Tirone, B.A., Kyle Possemato, Ph.D., and Robert Shoemaker of the Syracuse Veterans Affairs Hospital, for providing valuable editorial suggestions for this chapter.

1. Lang Divorce papers, 124/J/15/F, Minnesota State Archives, Minnesota Historical Society, Minneapolis, MN; source transcribed and published by Michael Schroeder: http://www.familyhistoryfiles.com/site_text/Documents/nellie_divorce_papers.htm (accessed March 5, 2009).

2. Frank Lang Compiled Service Record, National Archives and Record

Administration, Washington DC; source transcribed and published by Michael Schroeder: http://www.familyhistoryfiles.com/site_text/Documents/frankcivil-war.htm (accessed March 5, 2009)

3. Dave Grossman, *On Killing: The Psychological Cost of Learning to Kill in War and Society* (Boston: Little, Brown & Company, 1995), 367. There are several different listing of Frank Lang's age. His birth date (1842), places him to be age nineteen on enlistment in 1861. The role of enlisted men from Michigan's Company K recorded Frank Lang as age twenty-two in 1861. In this chapter, re-enlistment records were used to calculate his age because they are based on an actual declaration from Mr. Lang taken in December of 1863.

4. Andrew Carroll (ed.), *War Letters: Extraordinary Correspondence from American Wars* (New York: Scribner, 2001), 90-91.

5. Peter Kadzis (ed.), *Blood: Stories of Life and Death from the Civil War* (New York: Thunder's Mouth Press, 2000), 178-179, 187.

6. Lang Divorce papers.

7. Judith Herman, *Trauma and Recovery* (New York: Basic Books. 1997), 7-32; Drew Gilpin Faust, *This Republic of Suffering* (New York: Knopf, 2008), xi-xviii; Judith Pizarro, Roxane Cohen Silver, and JoAnn Prause, "Physical and Mental Health Costs of Traumatic War Experiences Among Civil War Veterans," *Archives of General Psychiatry*, 63 (Feb 2006), 193-200.

8. *Diagnostic and Statistical Manual of Mental Disorders*, Fourth Edition (Washington DC: American Psychiatric Association, 1994), 429-455

9. Lisa Long, *Rehabilitating Bodies: Health, History, and the American Civil War* (Philadelphia: University of Philadelphia Press, 2004), 1-28.

10. Albert Glass, "Army Psychiatry Through the Civil War," in *Psychiatry in the U.S. Army: Lessons for Community Psychiatry* (Wshington, DC: Defense Technical Information Center, 2005), 271; Herman, 20; Carol McMahon, "Nervous Disease and Malingering: The Status of Psychosomatic Concepts in Nineteenth Century Medicine," *International Journal of Psychosomatics*, 31 (1984), 15-19.

11. L. Swank and W. E. Marchand, "Combat Neuroses: Development of Combat Exhaustion, *Archives of Neurology and Psychology*,55 (1946): 236-47; Dave Grossman and Loren W. Christenson, *On Combat: The Psychology and Physiology of Deadly Conflict in War and in Peace* (Illinois: PPCT Research Publications, 2004), 12.

12. Glass, 2-25; Eric Dean, *Shook over Hell: Post-Traumatic Stress, Vietnam, and the Civil War* (Cambridge, MA: Harvard University Press, 1997), 70.

13. Robert Fogel, "Public Use Tape on the Aging of Veterans of the Union Army: Military, Pension, and Medical Records, 1860-1940," Version M-5 (Chicago: Center for Population Economics, University of Chicago Graduate School of Business and Provo, Utah: Department of Economics, Brigham Young University, 2000), 478; Robert Fogel, Public Use Tape on the Aging of Veterans of the Union Army: Surgeon's Certificates, 1862-1940," Version M-5 (Chicago: Center for Population Economics, University of Chicago Graduate School of Business and Provo, Utah: Department of Economics, Brigham Young University, 2001), 422.

14. Glass, 19-25

15. Herman, 21; Grossman, *On Killing*, 43-45.

16. Mable Deutrich, *Struggle for Supremacy: The Career of General Fred C. Ainsworth* (Washington: Public Affairs Press, 1962), 170; Fogel, "Public Use Tape on the Aging of Veterans of the Union Army: Surgeon's Certificates, 1862-1940."

17. Fogel, "Public Use Tape on the Aging of Veterans of the Union Army: Surgeon's Certificates, 1862-1940"; Fogel, "Public Use Tape on the Aging of Veterans of the Union Army: Military, Pension, and Medical Records, 1860-1940."

18. For a detailed review of the accuracy and completeness of the NIH funded transcription of Civil War records, see Pizarro, 193-200.

19. Ibid.

21. Roger K. Pitman, "Combat Effects on Mental Health," *Archives of General Psychiatry*, 63 (2006), 127-128.

21. Bruce Dohrenwend, et al., "The Psychological Risks of Vietnam for U.S. Veterans: A Revisit with New Data and Methods," *Science*, 313 (2006), 979-982; Zahava Solomon, "The Impact of Posttraumatic Stress Disorder in Military Situations," *Journal of Clinical Psychiatry*, 62 (2001), 11-15.

Bibliography

Archives
  Charleston, South Carolina
    Medical University of South Carolina Library
      Letters (1855-1862) of Francis Peyre Porcher
  Newberry, South Carolina
    Wessels Library, Newberry College
      Letter Book, Dr. J. J. Chisolm, Medical Purveyor, C.S.A., Columbia, S.C.
  Philadelphia, PA
    Library of the College of Physicians of Philadelphia
  Richmond, Virginia
    Virginia Commonwealth University
      Tompkins-McCaw Library Special Collections and Archives
        Sanger Historical Files
    Virginia Historical Society
      Grisgsby Family Papers
      Wickham Family Papers, 1766-1955
  Rockville, MD
    F. Terry Hambrecht Collection
  Washington, DC
    National Archives and Records Administration
      War Department Collection of Confederate Records
        Maj. A. Snowden Piggot Papers
        Medical Department
    United States Patent and Trademark Office

Newspapers
  American Presbyterian (Pittsburgh, PA)
  Burlington (IA) *Weekly Hawk-Eye*
  Charleston (SC) *Mercury*
  Daily Dispatch (Richmond, VA)
  Daily Morning Post (Philadelphia, PA)

Lancaster (PA) *Intelligencer*

Milwaukee Daily Sentinel

New York Times

Richmond (VA) *Enquirer*

Savannah (GA) *Republican*

Scientific American

Western Democrat (Charlotte, NC)

Books

The American Medical Ethics Revolution: How the AMA's Code of Ethics Has Transformed Physicians' Relationships to Patients, Professionals, and Society. Baltimore: John Hopkins University Press, 1999.

American National Biography. New York: Oxford Press, 1998.

Annual Report of the Commissioner of Patents for the Year 1865. Washington: Government Printing Office, 1867.

Bartholow, R. *A Manual of Instructions for Enlisting and Discharging Soldiers.* Philadelphia: J. B. Lippincott, 1863.

Blanton, W. B. *Medicine in Virginia in the Nineteenth Century.* Richmond: Garrett & Massie, 1933.

Boyle, C. J. (ed.) *Twice Remembered: Moments in the History of Spring Hill College.* Mobile: Friends of Spring Hill College Library, 1993.

Boutwell, G. S. *Reminiscences of Sixty Years in Public Affairs*, 2 vols. New York: McClure, Phillips, 1902.

Bragg, C. L., et al. *Never for Want of Powder: The Confederate Powder Works in Augusta, Georgia.* Columbia: University of South Carolina Press, 2007.

Burr, A. R., *Weir Mitchell: His Life and Letters.* New York, Duffield, 1929.

Butler, S. W. *The Medical Register and Directory of the United States.* Philadelphia: Office of the Medical and Surgical Reporter, 1874.

Calcutt, R. B. *Richmond's Wartime Hospitals.* Gretna, La: Pelican Publishing Company, 2005.

Carroll, A. (ed.) *War Letters: Extraordinary Correspondence from American Wars.* New York: Scribner, 2001.

Carson, J. *Synopsis of the Course of Lectures on Materia Medica and Pharmacy, Delivered in the University of Pennsylvania.* Philadelphia: Blanchard and Lea, 1855.

Catalogue of the Medical College of Virginia, Session 1862-1863. Richmond: Charles H. Wynne, 1863.

Catalogue of the Trustees, Officers, and Students of the University of Pennsylvania Session 1859-1860. Philadelphia: Collins, 1860.

Catalogue of the Officers, Students and Graduates of the Medical College of Virginia,

Session 1859-60 and Announcement of Session 1860-61. Richmond: Charles H. Wynne, 1860.

Catalogue of the Trustees, Officers, and Students of the University of Pennsylvania Session 1859-1860. Philadelphia: Collins, 1860.

The Centennial History of the Tennessee State Medical Association, 1830-1930. Nashville: Tennessee State Medical Association, 1930.

Chisolm, J.J. *A Manual of Military Surgery for the Use of Surgeons in the Confederate States Army*. Richmond, VA: West and Johnson, 1861.

Chisolm, J.J. *A Manual of Military Surgery for the Use of Surgeons in the Confederate States Army*. Richmond, VA: West and Johnson, 1862.

Chisolm, J. J. *A Manual of Military Surgery for the Use of Surgeons in the Confederate States Army*. Columbia, SC: Evans and Cogswell, 1864.

Cunningham, H.H. *Doctors in Gray: The Confederate Medical Service*. Baton Rouge: Louisiana State University Press, 1958.

Dean, E. *Shook over Hell: Post-Traumatic Stress, Vietnam, and the Civil War*. Cambridge, MA: Harvard University Press, 1997.

Deutrich, M., *Struggle for Supremacy: The Career of General Fred C. Ainsworth*. Washington: Public Affairs Press, 1962.

Diagnostic and Statistical Manual of Mental Disorders, Fourth Edition. Washington DC: American Psychiatric Association, 1994.

Dictionary of American Biography. New York: Charles Scribner's Sons, 1933.

Duffy, J. (ed.) *The Rudolph Matas History of Medicine in Louisiana*. Baton Rouge: Louisiana State University Press, 1962.

Duffy, J. *Tulane University Medical Center: One Hundred and Fifty Years of Medical Education*. Baton Rouge: Louisiana State University Press, 1984.

Earnest, E. S. *S. Weir Mitchell: Novelist and Physician*. Philadelphia: University of Pennsylvania, 1950.

Erichsen, J. *The Science and Art of Surgery*. Philadelphia: Blanchard and Lea, 1854.

Faust, D. G. *This Republic of Suffering*. New York: Knopf, 2008.

Finkelman, P. (ed.) *His Soul Goes Marching On: Responses to John Brown and the Harpers Ferry Raid*. Charlottesville: University Press of Virginia, 1994.

The First 125 Years of the Medical College of Virginia. Richmond, Va.: Medical College of Virginia, 1963.

Flint, A. F. (ed.) *Contributions Relating to the Causation and Prevention of Disease, and to Camp Diseases*. New York: Hurd and Houghton, 1867.

Franke, N. H. *Pharmaceutical Conditions and Drug Supply in the Confederacy*. Madison: American Institute of the History of Pharmacy, 1955.

Frost, H. R. *Outlines of a Course of Lectures on the Materia Medica, Designed for the Use of Students, Delivered at the Medical College of the State of South Carolina*, 5th Edition. James and Williams, 1858.

Gaillard, E. S. *The Medical and Surgical Lessons of the Late War*. Louisville: Louisville Journal, 1868.

Garrison, F. H. *An Introduction to the History of Medicine*. Philadelphia, W. B. Saunders, 1929.

General Directions for Collecting and Drying Medicinal Substances for the Vegetable Kingdom. Richmond: Surgeon General's Office, 1862.

Green, C.C. *Chimborazo: The Confederacy's Largest Hospital*. Knoxville: University of Tennessee Press, 2004.

Gross, S. D. *A Manual of Military Surgery*. Philadelphia: J. B. Lippincott, 1861.

Gross, S. D. *A System of Surgery*, Second Edition. Philadelphia: Blanchard and Lea, 1862.

Grossman, D. *On Killing: The Psychological Cost of Learning to Kill in War and Society*. Boston: Little, Brown & Company, 1995.

Grossman, D. and Loren W. Christenson. *On Combat: The Psychology and Physiology of Deadly Conflict in War and in Peace*. Illinois: PPCT Research Publications, 2004.

Herman, J. *Trauma and Recovery*. New York: Basic Books. 1997.

Kadzis, P. (ed.) *Blood: Stories of Life and Death from the Civil War*. New York: Thunder's Mouth Press, 2000.

Keen, W. W. *The Surgical Operations on President Cleveland in 1893*. Philadelphia: J. B. Lippincott, 1928.

Kelly, H. A. and Walter L. Burrage. *American Medical Biographies*. Baltimore: Norman Remington, 1920.

Kelly, H. A. and Walter L. Burrage. *Dictionary of American Medical Biography*. New York: D. Appleton, 1928.

King, D. *Quackery Unmasked: Or a Consideration of the Most Prominent Empirical Schemes of the Present Time, with an Enumeration of Some of the Causes Which Contribute to Their Support*. Boston: David Clapp, 1858.

Koonce, D. B. (ed.) *Doctor to the Front: The Recollections of Confederate Surgeon Thomas Fanning Wood, 1861-1865*. Knoxville: University of Tennessee Press, 2000.

Lande, R. G. *Madness, Malingering, and Malfeasance*. Washington: Brassey's, 2003.

Letterman, J. *Medical Recollections of the Army of the Potomac*. New York: D. Appleton, 1866.

Lipman, J. *Rufus Porter: Yankee Pioneer*. New York: C.N. Potter, 1968.

Lohmeyer, C. F. *Die Schusswunden und ihre Behandlung Kurz bearb*. Gottingen: Wigand, 1859.

Long, L. *Rehabilitating Bodies: Health, History, and the American Civil War.* Philadelphia: University of Philadelphia Press, 2004.

Longmore, T. A. *Treatise on Gunshot Wounds.* Philadelphia: J. B. Lippincott, 1862.

MacLeod, G.H.B. *Notes on the Surgery of the War in the Crimea With Remarks on the Treatment of Gunshot Wounds.* Philadelphia: JB Lippincott, 1862.

Massey, M. E. *Ersatz in the Confederacy.* Columbia: University of South Carolina Press, 1993.

McHenry, L. C. *Garrison's History of Neurology.* Springfield, MA: Charles C. Thomas, 1969.

McPherson, J. M., *Battle Cry of Freedom: The Civil War Era.* New York: Oxford University Press, 2003.

Medical and Surgical History of the British Army Which Served in Turkey and the Crimea During the War Against Russia in the Years 1854-55-56. London, 1858.

The Medical and Surgical History of the War of the Rebellion. Washington, DC: Government Printing Office, 1888.

Mitchell, J. K. *Remote Consequences of Injuries of Nerves and their Treatment.* Philadelphia: Lea Brothers, 1895.

Mitchell, S. W. *Injuries of Nerves and Their Consequences.* Philadelphia: J. B. Lippincott, 1872.

Mitchell, S. W. *In War Time.* Boston: Houghton Mifflin, 1885.

Mitchell, S. W. *Researches upon the Venom of the Rattlesnake.* Washington: Smithsonian, 1861.

Mitchell, S. W., G. R. Morehouse, W. W. Keen. *Gunshot Wounds and Other Injuries of Nerves.* Philadelphia: J. B. Lippincott, 1864.

Mitchell, S. W., G. R. Morehouse, W. W. Keen. *Gunshot Wounds and Other Injuries of Nerves,* Reprint with Biographical Introduction by Ira M. Rutkow. San Francisco: Norman, 1989.

Mitchell, S. W., G. R. Morehouse, W. W. Keen. *Reflex Paralysis,* Circular No. 6. Washington: Surgeon General's Office, 1864.

Mitchell, S. W., G. R. Morehouse, W. W. Keen. *Reflex Paralysis,* Circular No. 6, Reprint with Introduction by John F. Fulton. New Haven: Yale University School of Medicine, 1941.

The National Cyclopedia of American Biography. New York: James T. White, 1906.

Norwood, W. F. *Medical Education in the United States Before the Civil War.* New York: Arno Press, 1971.

Nosworthy, B. *The Bloody Crucible of Courage: Fighting Methods and Combat Experience of the Civil War.* Berkeley, CA: Carroll & Graf, 2003.

Officers of the MCV Session 1853-1854 Announcement of the Session 1854-1855. Richmond, VA, 1854.

Olnhausen, M.P. *Adventures of an Army Nurse in Two Wars*. Boston: Little Brown, 1903.

Pace, R. F. *Halls of Honor: College Men in the Old South*. Baton Rouge: Louisiana State University Press, 2004.

Parish, P. J. *The American Civil War*. New York: Holmes and Meier, 1975.

The Pharmacopoeia of the United States of America. Boston: Wells and Lilly, 1820.

Porcher, F. P. *Resources of the Southern Fields and Forests, Medical, Economical, and Agricultural*. Charleston: Evans & Cogswell, 1863.

Porcher, F. P. *Resources of the Southern Fields and Forests, Medical, Economical, and Agricultural*, Reprint with Biographical Introduction by Ira M. Rutkow. San Francisco: Norman Publishing, 1991.

Psychiatry in the U.S. Army: Lessons for Community Psychiatry. Washington, DC: Defense Technical Information Center, 2005.

Reed, W. H. *Hospital Life in the Army of the Potomac*. Boston: William V. Spencer, 1866.

Regulations for the Army of the Confederate States, 1862. Richmond: J. W. Randolph, 1862.

Regulations for the Medical Department of the C.S. Army. Richmond, Richie & Dunnavant, 1863.

Rothstein, W. G. *American Medical Schools and the Practice of Medicine*. New York: Oxford University Press, 1989.

Rutkow, I. M. *The History of Surgery in the United States, 1775-1900*. San Francisco: Norman, 1988.

Schmidt, J. M. *Lincoln's Labels: America's Best Known Brands and the Civil War*. Roseville, MN: Edinborough Press, 2008.

Spaulding, P. *The History of the Medical College of Georgia*. Athens: University of Georgia Press, 1987.

Standard Supply Table of the Indigenous Remedies for Field Service and the Sick in General Hospitals. Richmond: Surgeon General's Office, 1863.

Stromeyer, L. *Maximen der Kriegsheilkunst*. Hanover, 1855.

S. Weir Mitchell, 1828-1914, Memorial Addresses and Resolutions. Philadelphia: College of Physicians of Philadelphia, 1914.

Tanner, R. G. *Stonewall in the Valley: Thomas J. "Stonewall" Jackson's Shenandoah Valley Campaign, Spring 1862*. Garden City, NY: Doubleday, 1976.

Taylor, F. H. *Philadelphia in the Civil War, 1861-1865*. Philadelphia: City of Philadelphia, 1913.

Taylor, Mrs. T. and S. E. Conner (eds.) *South Carolina Women in the Confederacy*, Vol. 1. Columbia: State Company, 1903.

Transactions of the Ninth Annual Meeting of the Ohio State Medical Society. Cincinnati: West American Monthly, 1854.

Travis, J. *Wounded Hearts: Masculinity, Law, and Literature in American Culture.* Chapel Hill: University of North Carolina Press, 2005.

Tripler, C. S. and G. C. Blackman. *Handbook for the Military Surgeon.* Cincinnati: Robert Clarke, 1861.

Tucker, B. R. *Tales of the Tuckers: Descendents of the Male Line of St. George Tucker.* Richmond: The Dietz Printing Company, 1941.

Vandiver, F. E. *Ploughshares into Swords: Josiah Gorgas and Confederate Ordnance.* College Station: Texas A&M University Press, 1994.

Waring, J. I. *A History of Medicine in South Carolina 1825-1900.* Columbia: South Carolina Medical Association, 1967.

Walter, R. D. *S. Weir Mitchell, M. D.—Neurologist.* Springfield, MA: Charles C. Thomas, 1970.

The War of the Rebellion: A Compilation of the Official Records of the Union and Confederate Armies. Washington: Government Printing Office, 1880-1901.

Westmoreland, J. G. *A Syllabus of Lectures on Materia Medica and Therapeutics, Delivered in the Atlanta Medical College.* Atlanta: G. P. Eddy, 1857.

Wood, G. B. and F. Bache. *The Dispensatory of the United States of America.* Philadelphia: J. B. Lippincott, 1858.

Woodrow, M. W. (ed.) *Dr. James Woodrow as Seen by His Friends.* Columbia: R. L. Bryan, 1909.

Worthington, C. F., C. F, and H. Adams. *A Cycle of Adams Letters*, 2 vols. Boston: Houghton Mifflin, 1920.

Women Inventors to Whom Patents Have Been Granted by the United States Government, 1790-1895. Washington: Government Printing Office, 1895.

Zajtchuk, R. and Ronald F. Bellamy (eds.) *Medical Aspects of Chemical and Biological Warfare.* Washington, D.C.: Office of the Surgeon General of the Army, 1997.

Articles

Abrahams, H. J. "Secession from Northern Medical Schools." *Transactions and Studies of the College of Physicians of Philadelphia*, Vol. 36, July 1968, 29-45.

"Association of Army and Navy Surgeons." *Confederates States Medical and Surgical Journal*, Vol. 1, January 1864, 13-16.

Berman, A. "Striving for Scientific Respectability: Some American Botanics and the Nineteenth-Century Plant Materia Medica." *Bulletin of the History of Medicine*, Vol. 30, January-February 1956, 7-31.

Bigelow, H. J. "Urethral Catheters." *Boston Medical and Surgical Journal*, Vol. 40, 1849, 9.

Bowers, R. V. "Civil War Days at the Medical College of Virginia." *The Scarab*, Vol. 10, August 1961, 1-3.

Bowers, R. V. "Our Faculty in Gray—MCV 1860-1861." *The Scarab*, Vol. 13, February 1964, 1-4.

Breeden, J. O. "Medical Shortages and Confederate Medicine: A Retrospective Evaluation." *Southern Medical Journal*, Vol. 86, September 1993, 1040-48.

Breeden, J. O. "States-rights Medicine in the Old South." *Bulletin of the New York Academy of Medicine*, Vol. 52, March-April 1976, 348-72.

Calhoun, J. T. "Rough Notes of an Army Surgeon's Experience During the Great Rebellion." *Medical and Surgical Reporter*, Vol. 9, 1862, 303.

Canale, D. J. "Civil War Medicine from the Perspective of S. Weir Mitchell's 'The Case of George Dedlow.'" *Journal of the History of the Neurosciences*, Vol. 13, 2004, 7-21.

Caniff, W. "Surgery of the Federal Army." *Lancet*, Vol. 1, 1863, 251-2.

Carpenter, C. H. "Fatal Kidney Injuries." *Boston Medical and Surgical Journal*, Vol. 71, 1865, 112.

"The Case of George Dedlow." *The Atlantic Monthly*, July 1866, 1-11.

Dohrenwend, B., et al. "The Psychological Risks of Vietnam for U.S. Veterans: A Revisit with New Data and Methods." *Science*, Vol. 313, 2006, 979-982.

Dougherty, P. J. and H. C. Eidt. "Wound Ballistics: Minie ball vs. full Metal Jacketed Bullets—A Comparison of Civil War and Spanish-American War Firearms." *Military Medicine*, Vol. 174, 2009, 403-407.

Duffy, J. "Sectional Conflict and Medical Education in Louisiana." *Journal of Southern History*, Vol. 23, August 1957, 303.

Dusenbury, H. "Cases of Gunshot Wounds of the Abdomen Involving Viscera." *American Journal of the Medical Sciences*, Vol. 50 , 1865, 400.

"Editorial and Miscellaneous." *Virginia Medical and Surgical Journal*, Vol. 3, April 1854, 86-88.

Flynt, W. "Southern Higher Education and the Civil War." *Civil War History*, Vol. 14, June 1968, 211-225.

Freemon, F. R. "Detecting Feigned Illness During the American Civil War." *Journal of the History of the Neurosciences*, Vol. 2, 1993, 239-41.

Freemon, F. R. "The First Neurological Research Center: Turner's Lane Hospital During the American Civil War." *Journal of the History of the Neurosciences*, Vol. 2, 1993, 135-42.

Frost, H. R. "Cotton Seed (Gossypium Herbaceum) as an Antiperiodic in Intermittent Fever." *Charleston Medical Journal and Review*, Vol. 5, 1850, 416.

Fulton, J. F., "Medicine, Warfare, and History." *Journal of the American Medical Association*, Vol. 153, 1953, 482-88.

Fulton, J. F. "Neurology and War." *Transactions and Studies of the College of Physicians*, Vol. 8, 1940, 157-65.

Fye, W. B. "S. Weir Mitchell, Philadelphia's 'Lost Physiologist.'" *Bulletin of the History of Medicine*, Vol. 57, 1983, 188-202.

Goetz, C. G. and M. J. Aminoff. "The Brown-Sequard and S. Weir Mitchell Letters." *Neurology*, Vol. 57, 2100-2104.

Goetz, C. G. "Jean-Martin Charcot and Silas Weir Mitchell." *Neurology*, Vol. 48, 1997, 1128-32.

Griliches, Z. "Patent Statistics as Economic Indicators: A Survey." *Journal of Economic Literature*, Vol. 28, December 1990, 1661-1707.

Hambrecht, F. T., M. Rhode, and A. Hawk. "Dr. Chisolm's Inhaler: A Rare Confederate Medical Invention." *The Journal of the South Carolina Medical Association*, Vol. 87, May 1991, 277-280.

Hamilton, F. H. "Gunshot Wounds of the Penis." *American Medical Times*, Vol. 9, 1864, 61.

Hamilton, F. H. "Gunshot Wounds of the Scrotum and Testes." *American Medical Times*, Vol. 9, 1864, 61.

Hasegawa, G. R. "'Absurd Prejudice': A. Snowden Piggot and the Confederate Medical Laboratory at Lincolnton." *North Carolina Historical Review*, Vol. 81, July 2004, 313-34.

Hasegawa, G. R. "Proposals for chemical weapons during the American Civil War." *Military Medicine*, Vol. 173, May 2008, 499-506.

Hasegawa, G. R. "Quinine Substitutes in the Confederate Army." *Military Medicine*, Vol. 172, June 2007, 650-55.

Hasegawa, G. R. "Confederate Medical Purveying in Savannah and Macon." Presentation at the Thirteenth Annual Conference on Civil War Medicine, Hagerstown, MD, 10 Oct 2005.

Hasegawa, G. R. and F. T. Hambrecht "The Confederate Medical Laboratories." *Southern Medical Journal*, Vol. 96, December 2003, 1221-30.

Homans, J. "Gunshot Wounds of the Testes." *Boston Medical and Surgical Journal*, Vol. 72, 1865, 15.

Jacobs, J. "Some of the Drug Conditions during the War Between the States, 1861-1865." *Proceedings of the American Pharmaceutical Association*, Vol. 46, 1898, 192-213.

Jones, J. "Indigenous Remedies of the Southern Confederacy Which May Be Employed in the Treatment of Malarial Fever." *Southern Medical and Surgical Journal*, Vol. 17, September -October 1861, 673-718, 753-87.

"Karl Theodor Mohr: Eine Biographische Skizze." *Pharmaceutische Rundschau*, Vol. 5, February 1887, 4-12.

Keen, W. W., S. W. Mitchell, and G. R. Morehouse. "On Malingering, Especially in Regard to Simulation of Diseases of the Nervous System." *American Journal of the Medical Sciences*, Vol. 48, 1864, 367-94.

Keen, W.W. "Surgical Reminiscences of the Civil War." *Transactions of the College of Physicians of Philadelphia*, Third Series, Vol. 27, 1905, 95-114.

Kennedy, S. "Turpentine as a Remedial Agent." *Medical and Surgical Reporter*, Vol. 16, 1 June 1867, 458-59.

Khan, Z. B., "'Not for Ornament': Patenting Activity by Nineteenth-Century Women Inventors." *Journal of Interdisciplinary History*, Vol. 31, Autumn 2000, 159-95.

Kilbride, D. "Southern Medical Students in Philadelphia, 1800-1861: Science and Sociability in the 'Republic of Medicine.'" *Journal of Southern History*, Vol. 65, November 1999, 697-732.

Levin, A. "Civil War Trauma Led to Combination of Nervous and Physical Disease." *Psychiatric News*, Vol. 41, 2006, 2.

Lewis, S. E. "Samuel Preston Moore, M.D., Surgeon General of the Confederate States." *Southern Practitioner*, Vol. 23, 1901, 381-86.

Lidell, J. A. "Injuries of Abdominal Viscera by Firearms. *American Journal of the Medical Sciences*, Vol. 53, 1867, 356.

MacLeod, C. "The Springs of Invention and British Industrialization." *Recent Findings of Research in Economic & Social History*, Spring 1995, 1-4.

Maisch, J. M. "Report on the Drug Market." *Proceedings of the American Pharmaceutical Association*, Vol. 12, 1864, 187-200.

McGuire, H. "Annual Address of the President." *Transactions of the Southern Surgical and Gynecological Association*, Vol. 2, 1890, 1-12.

McMahon, C. "Nervous Disease and Malingering: The Status of Psychosomatic Concepts in Nineteenth Century Medicine." *International Journal of Psychosomatics*, Vol. 31, 1984, 15-19.

"Medical Colleges of the United States." *Transactions of the American Medical Association*, 1848, 293.

Middleton, W. S. "The Fielding H. Garrison Lecture: Turner's Lane Hospital." *Bulletin of the History of Medicine*, Vol. 40, 1966, 14-42.

Mitchell, S. W. "Phantom Limbs." *Lippincott's Magazine of Popular Literature and Science*, Vol. 8, 1871, 563-69.

Mitchell, S. W. "Some Personal Recollections of the Civil War." *Transactions of the College of Physicians of Philadelphia*, Vol. 27, 1905, 87-94.

Moore, S. P. "Address of the President of the Association of Medical Officers of the Confederate States Army and Navy." *Southern Practitioner*, Vol. 31, October 1909, 491-98.

Moser, P. "How Do Patent Laws Influence Innovation? Evidence from

19th-Century World's Fairs." *American Economic Review*, Vol. 95, September 2005, 1215-1236.

Murrell, T. W. "The Exodus of Medical Students from Philadelphia, December, 1859." *Bulletin of the Medical College of Virginia*, Vol. 51, July 1954, 2-15.

"On the External Application of Oil of Turpentine as a Substitute for Quinine in Intermittent Fever, with Reports of Cases." *Confederate States Medical and Surgical Journal*, Vol. 1, January 1864, 7-8.

Pitman, R. K. "Combat Effects on Mental Health." *Archives of General Psychiatry*, Vol. 63, 2006, 127-128.

Pizarro, J., R. C. Silver, and J. Prause. "Physical and Mental Health Costs of Traumatic War Experiences Among Civil War Veterans." *Archives of General Psychiatry*, Vol. 63, February 2006, 193-200.

Porcher, F. P. "Report on the Indigenous Medicinal Plants of South Carolina." *Transactions of the American Medical Association*, Vol. 2, 1849, 667-862.

Porcher, F. P. "Resources of the Southern Fields and Forests." *De Bow's Review*, Vol. 6, New Series, August 1861, 105-31.

Porcher, F. P. "Suggestions Made to the Medical Department. Modifications of Treatment Required in the Management of the Confederate Soldier, Dependent upon His Peculiar Moral and Physical Condition; with a Reference to Certain Points in Practice." *Southern Medical and Surgical Journal*, Vol. 1, Series 3, September 1866, 248-86.

Porter, J. B. "Surgical Notes of the Mexican War." *American Journal of the Medical Sciences*, Vol. 23, 1852, 30.

"Professor James H. Conway.," *Confederate States Medical and Surgical Journal*, Vol. 2, February 1865, 39.

Ramsay, H. A. "Cotton Seed in Intermittent Fever." *Nashville Medical Journal*, Vol. 1, 1854, 150-51.

Riley, H. D. "Confederate Medical Manuals of the Civil War." *J. Med Assoc Ga*, Vol. 77, February 1988, 104-8.

"Salutatory." *Confederates States Medical and Surgical Journal*, Vol. 1, January 1864, 13-16.

Sherman, R. "Julian John Chisolm, M.D.: President's Address." *The American Surgeon*, Vol. 55, January 1986, 1-8.

Solomon, Z. "The Impact of Posttraumatic Stress Disorder in Military Situations." *Journal of Clinical Psychiatry*, Vol. 62, 2001, 11-15.

"Staff of the Southern Reform Medical College." *Southern Medical Reformer & Review*, Vol. 9 March 1859, p. 1.

Stone, J. L. "W. W. Keen: America's Pioneer Neurological Surgeon." *Neurosurgery*, Vol. 17, 1985, 997-1010.

Swank, L. and W. E. Marchand. "Combat Neuroses: Development of Combat Exhaustion," *Archives of Neurology and Psychology*, Vol. 55, 1946, 236-47.

Taylor, W. H. "Some Experiences of a Confederate Assistant Surgeon." *Transactions of the College of Physicians of Philadelphia*, Vol. 28, Third Series, 1906, 91-121.

Townsend, J. M. "Francis Peyre Porcher, M.D." *Annals of Medical History*, Vol. 1, Third Series, 1939, 177-88.

Trent, P. "Intermittent Fever Treated by Decoction of Gossypium herbaceum, or Cotton-Seed." *Charleston Medical Journal and Review*, Vol. 9, 1854, 97-98.

Warner, J. H. "A Southern Medical Reform: The Meaning of the Antebellum Argument for Southern Medical Education." *Bulletin of the History of Medicine*, Vol. 57, Fall 1983, 364-81.

Manuscripts and Databases
Borut, M. "The *Scientific American* in Nineteenth Century America." unpublished Ph.D. dissertation. New York: New York University, 1977.

Duncan, L. C. *The Medical Department of the United States Army in the Civil War* n.p., n.d.

Dwyer, J. L. "Adult Education in Civil War Richmond January 1861-April 1865." Unpublished EdD disseratation. Blacksburg, VA: Virginia Polytechnic Institute and State University, 1997.

Fogel, R. "Public Use Tape on the Aging of Veterans of the Union Army: Military, Pension, and Medical Records, 1860-1940," Version M-5. Chicago: Center for Population Economics, University of Chicago Graduate School of Business and Provo, Utah: Department of Economics, Brigham Young University, 2000.

Fogel, R. "Public Use Tape on the Aging of Veterans of the Union Army: Surgeon's Certificates, 1862-1940," Version M-5. Chicago: Center for Population Economics, University of Chicago Graduate School of Business and Provo, Utah: Department of Economics, Brigham Young University, 2001.

Gustafson, R. "A Study of the Life of James Woodrow Emphasizing His Theological and Scientific View as They Relate to the Evolution Controversy." Unpublished Ph.D. dissertation. Richmond, VA: Union Theological Seminary, 1964.

MacLeod, C. and A. Nuvolari "Inventive Activities, Patents and Early Industrialization: A Synthesis of Research Issues." Danish Research Institute for Industrial Dynamics (DRUID) Working Paper 06-28, 2006.

"Seaman Prize Essay—The Comparative Mortality of Disease and Battle Casualties in the Historic Wars of the World." n.p, c. 1910.

Stampp, K. M. (ed.) "Records of Ante-Bellum Southern Plantations from the Revolution through the Civil War," Microfilm. Bethesda: University Publications of America, n.d.

Index

About the Authors

James M. Schmidt

James M. Schmidt is a bioanalytical chemist by training and profession. After receiving his B.S. in Chemistry from the University of Central Oklahoma, he has worked in a number of private, government, and industrial laboratories, and is currently employed as a research scientist with a biotech firm in The Woodlands, Texas.

Mr. Schmidt has had a life-long interest in military history, with a special regard for the Civil War. His historical writing credits include articles for *North & South*, *The Artilleryman*, *World War II*, *Learning Through History*, *Today's Chemist*, and *Chemical Heritage* magazines. His column, "Medical Department," has appeared regularly in *The Civil War News* since 2000. He has also given lectures on the Civil War to groups in Ohio, Missouri, Illinois, Tennessee, and Texas.

Mr. Schmidt's first book, *Lincoln's Labels: America's Best Known Brands and the Civil War*, was published by Edinborough Press in Spring 2008.

Guy R. Hasegawa, Pharm.D.

Dr. Guy R. Hasegawa is Senior Editor of the *American Journal of Health-System Pharmacy* (Bethesda, MD). He received a B.A. in Zoology from the University of California, Los Angeles, and a Doctor of Pharmacy degree from the University of California, San Francisco, before completing a hospital-pharmacy residency at the University of Illinois at Chicago. Before moving to Maryland, he was a clinical pharmacist at St. Joseph Mercy Hospital, Ann Arbor, MI, and Clinical Assistant Professor at the University of Michigan College of Pharmacy.

Dr. Hasegawa's interest in writing, the Civil War, and medicine has led to his publication of historical articles in various scholarly periodicals, including the *American Journal of Health-System Pharmacy*, the *Journal of the American College of Surgeons*, *Military Medicine*, the *North Carolina Historical Review*, and the *Southern Medical Journal*. His primary Civil War interests are drug therapy, medical purveying, and pharmacy. He has lectured frequently at conferences of the National Museum of Civil War Medicine and the Society of Civil War Surgeons and serves on the board of directors of both organizations.

Judith Andersen, Ph.D.

Dr. Judith Andersen is an experimental psychologist by training and profession. She received her Ph.D. in psychology from the University of California, Irvine in 2007. Specializing in health psychology, she has focused her research on the physical and mental health outcomes of traumatic and stressful experience. After graduate school, she spent time as a faculty member in the Department of Psychology at Syracuse University, and served as a Research Scientist at the Veterans Affairs Hospital in Syracuse, New York. Dr. Andersen is currently a Post-Doctoral Fellow in the Psychology Department at Cornell University.

In addition to conducting research on the health outcomes of exposure to September 11th, 2001, Dr. Andersen has pursued a long standing interest in military medicine by completing an in-depth analysis of the mental and physical health of Civil War veterans. Her writing credits include empirical articles published in the *Archives of General Psychiatry*, *Health Psychology*, and the *Journal of Aggression, Maltreatment & Trauma*, among others.

Alfred Jay Bollet, M.D.

Dr. Alfred Jay Bollet has been a lifelong student of all aspects of the Civil War, and has studied the medical history of the war intensively for over a dozen years. Born in New York City and a graduate of New York University, he spent his professional career in academic medicine, serving as a professor of internal medicine at the University of Virginia, the Medical College of Georgia, and State University of New York at Brooklyn. He was chairman of the Department of Medicine at the latter two institutions.

Recently, he has been Clinical Professor of Medicine at Yale. Dr. Bollet, now retired, has published numerous papers and presented lectures on various aspects of Civil War medicine at many medical schools, Civil War Round Tables, and the Smithsonian Institution. He serves on the Honorary Board of Advisors of the National Museum of Civil War Medicine in Frederick, Maryland, and is on the Board of Directors of the Society of Civil War Surgeons.

Dr. Bollet is the author of the acclaimed book, *Civil War Medicine: Challenges and Triumphs*, which was a selection of the History Book Club and received the writing prize of the Army Historical Foundation for 2002 (the first book on a medical topic to receive the prize).

D.J. Canale, M.D.

Dr. D. J. Canale has had a distinguished career as a surgeon and a medical historian. He graduated from the University of Tennessee College of Medicine in 1955, and performed postgraduate training and internships in neurosurgery at Henry Ford Hospital in Detroit. He served three years in the United States Air Force as a Flight Surgeon.

Dr. Canale served as president of the Memphis and Shelby County medical societies, was recently president of the American Osler Society, and is currently historian of the Southern Neurosurgical Society.

In the past few years, Dr. Canale has devoted particular attention to studying Civil War medicine. He is the author of more than a dozen articles on the history of medicine, with publications in the *Journal of the History of Neuroscience, Tennessee Medicine, Neurosurgery*, and many others.

F. Terry Hambrecht, M.D.

F. Terry Hambrecht, M.D., is a co-founder of the National Museum of Civil War Medicine in Frederick, Maryland. He republished and updated two nineteen-century books, one on Union regimental physicians and the other on Civil War medical instruments, and has written several original papers on Civil War medicine. For the past twenty years he has been preparing a biographical register of physicians who served the Confederacy in a medical capacity.

Trained as an electrical engineer and a physician, he retired from the National Institutes of Health (NIH) where he spent over 30 years both in the laboratory and as the director of NIH's international program for developing implantable neural prostheses. Among these were the multichannel cochlear implant for hearing impaired and an implanted functional neuromuscular stimulation system for paralyzed individuals. Both of these neural prostheses have been approved by the FDA and are commercially available.

Dr. Hambrecht currently enjoys research on Civil War medicine, modeling O gauge electric trains, enabling individuals with physical disabilities to utilize technology for interacting with their environment, and travel with his wife, Maureen.

Harry Herr, M.D.

Dr. Harry Herr is an academic urologic surgeon by profession. After receiving A.B (Biology) and M.D. degress from the University of California, he completed specialty training in urology and oncology at the Sloan-Kettering Insitute for Cancer Research and Cornell. He is currently an Attending Surgeon in the Department of Urology at the Memorial Sloan-Kettering Cancer Center and Professor of Urology at Cornell Medical College in New York.

Dr. Herr holds a life-long interest in the history of science and medicine, with special regard for the evolution of surgery. Contributing numerous articles to medical and historical journals, many of which highlight medical care during the Civil War, he established and serves as Editor of the History Section of the *Journal of Urology*.

Dr. Herr is an avid historian and frequent participant in history seminars, while maintaining an active surgical and research practice in urologic oncology.

Jodi Koste

Jodi Koste began working at Tompkins-McCaw Library for the Health Sciences in March of 1978. She holds a B.A. and M.A. in History from Old Dominion University. Since 1981 she has served as Archivist for the Medical College of Virginia Campus and has been actively involved in promoting and preserving the documentary heritage of the institution. She has taught semester long classes in archival administration for Virginia Commonwealth University and the University of Mary Washington. She is an active member of the American Association for the History of Medicine, Archivists and Librarians in the History of the Health Sciences, the Society of American Archivists and the Mid-Atlantic Regional Archives Conference.

Ms. Koste's work has appeared in *American National Biography*, *Dictionary of Virginia Biography*, *Jewish Women in America: a Historical Encyclopedia*, and *Encyclopedia of the Confederacy*.